RENEWALS: 691-4574

DATE DUE

DEC 17			
ILL. 2847232 AHH			NO RENEWALS OCT 0 1 1994
MAR 1 1			
MAR 2 6			
APR 2 2			
MAY 6			

Demco, Inc. 38-293

Orphan Drugs

Orphan Drugs

Medical versus Market Value

Carolyn H. Asbury
University of Pennsylvania

Lexington Books
D.C. Heath and Company/Lexington, Massachusetts/Toronto

Library of Congress Cataloging in Publication Data

Asbury, Carolyn H.
  Orphan drugs.

  Includes index.
  1. Pharmaceutical policy—United States.   2. Drug
trade—United States.   I. Title.   [DNLM: 1. Drug Industry
—economics—United States.   2. Drugs.   3. Legislation,
Drug—United States.   4. Public Policy—United States.
QV 736 A799o]
RA401.A3A83   1985   362.1'782   84–47648
ISBN 0–669–08389–5 (alk. paper)

Published simultaneously in Canada
Printed in the United States of America on acid-free paper
International Standard Book Number: 0–669–08389–5
Library of Congress Catalog Card Number: 84–47648

To Arthur K. Asbury, M.D.
Who encouraged, advised, and sustained

Contents

List of Figure and Tables

Foreword

After a long period of neglect, issues concerning orphan drugs are finally receiving the attention they deserve. Dr. Carolyn Asbury's research provides the first in-depth, systematic analysis of orphan drugs, which affect the health of millions of Americans, as well as most of the world's population. Dr. Asbury has carried out a detailed review and analysis of the literature on the subject; she has conducted a series of interviews with top industry people and federal agency officials; and she has collaborated with the staff of the Subcommittee on Health and the Environment, U.S. House of Representatives, in conducting a survey of 121 drugs of limited commercial interest and analyzing the data generated from that survey. In fact, Dr. Asbury's research contributed to the development of the first federal legislation on orphan drugs, providing not only new information but also a framework for examining policy issues related to orphan drugs and for evaluating the effects of legislation in this field.

In this very stimulating and valuable book, Dr. Asbury examines the problems attending orphan drugs within the overall context of the evolution of drug development, approval, and marketing in the United States during the past several decades. She also examines congressional rationale for and potential strengths and weaknesses of legislation in this area. In addition, she addresses important ethical and public-policy issues.

This book is an important contribution to an understanding of prescription drugs and prescription drug policies in the United States. It should be a valuable resource not only to policymakers in the Food and Drug Administration of the Department of Health and Human Services and other federal agencies, but also to policymakers in the drug industry, in international agencies, in other industrialized nations, and in Third World countries.

Philip R. Lee, M.D.
Professor of Social Medicine
Director, Institute for Health
  Policy Studies
University of California
San Francisco

Preface

Back in the late 1970s I first became aware of the problems confronting *orphan* (medically important but unprofitable) drugs, while working on a master's degree in public health at the Johns Hopkins School of Hygiene and Public Health. The drugs seemed to have fallen into the cracks of a highly complex and sophisticated system intended to bring medical drugs to those who need them. Federal efforts to develop plans and policies for these orphan drugs became the subject of the master's thesis.

During the next few years, while completing doctoral studies at the Wharton School, University of Pennsylvania, I began to use the tools of the systems approach to synthesize views from public health with those from the business of health. Public- and private-sector activities on orphan drugs were just evolving. Interviews with top officials in the industry and the government gave a new insight into the issues surrounding orphan drugs. During the course of these interviews, the opportunity arose to conduct jointly with the House Subcommittee on Health and the Environment, chaired by Representative Henry Waxman (D-Calif.), a survey of orphan drugs that had been identified by pharmaceutical industry and federal research agency sponsors.

Our purpose was to determine whether specific legislative measures might lessen regulatory and market obstructions and thereby increase industry willingness to develop and bring technically feasible orphan drugs to the market. At about the same time, the opportunity arose to participate in planning efforts as an invited (unpaid) consultant to the newly established Pharmaceutical Manufacturers Association Commission on Drugs for Rare Diseases. Much of the information in this book derives from these opportunities, from the active network of people in voluntary health organizations and academic research centers, and from members of the newly organized Food and Drug Administration (FDA) Office of Orphan Products Development.

Much of the information on orphan drugs contained in this book would probably never have been available without the firm commitment to the problems of those drugs demonstrated by Representative Waxman, and without the tremendous effort expended on the survey by William Corr, subcommittee counsel.

The orphan-drug survey was funded in part by generous grants from the Leonard Davis Institute of Health Economics at the Wharton School, a private University of Pennsylvania donor, and from the University of California, San Francisco, Institute for Health Policy Studies, directed by Philip R. Lee. He and I had planned to conduct an orphan-drug survey as part of a postdoctoral fellow research year at the UCSF institute the following year but the timing of the subcommittee's efforts required a change in those plans. At his urging, this book was begun during that year (1982–1983) and completed after return to the University of Pennsylvania as a senior fellow at the Leonard Davis Institute of Health Economics.

The efforts of many people were invaluable throughout this project. Top industry officials from seven major firms generously gave their time, expertise and insights during interviews (and, because they were promised anonymity, they must go nameless here). Additionally, John Eckman, chairman of the board and chief executive officer of Rorer Group, Inc., and past chairman of the board of the PMA, was especially helpful in facilitating my participation with the PMA commission, as were the commission's John Adams and Theodore Cooper.

Top officials from federal research and regulatory agencies (also granted anonymity) were similarly helpful in providing valuable information and perspective on the problems they face with orphan drugs.

Guidance and aid in the research came from many in academia, most notably Paul Stolley, William Kissick, Samuel Martin III (all from the medical school), and Russell Ackoff, Thomas Cowan, Hasan Ozbekhan, Larry Hirschhorn, Robert Graham and Robert Inman (all from the Wharton School) at the University of Pennsylvania; and from USCF, Philip R. Lee, and Jere Goyan, dean of the School of Pharmacy and former FDA Commissioner.

Finally, this book has had the benefit of expert editing. Ruth and Charles Holstein, whose careers in the executive and legislative branches of government have provided them with firsthand knowledge of much of the legislation discussed in the book, breathed life and accuracy into its chapters. Finally, Arthur K. Asbury, M.D., my husband, lent his medical and literary expertise through fastidious editing, which helped immeasurably to craft the final version presented here. Editor Kathryn Geiger and the staff at Lexington Books provided expert assistance throughout the process. To all these people, I am deeply indebted.

Orphan Drugs

1
What Makes Some Drugs Orphans?

Melvin Van Woert sat at his laboratory table at Mount Sinai School of Medicine, repeatedly measuring dosages of the shelf chemical 1–5HTP and encapsulating them in drug form. In the late 1970s and early 1980s, this experimental therapy was the only treatment available for his several patients with postanoxic myoclonus. This rare condition, caused by a critical period of oxygen deprivation, leaves patients with permanent neurological damage, causing shocklike muscle contractions.

Similarly, John Walshe, in his laboratory at the University of Cambridge, was purifying and packing into capsules the industrial solvent triethylene tetramine (trien) to use as a substitute drug for a nine-year-old boy and six other patients with life-threatening Wilsons disease, a disorder of copper metabolism. These few patients being treated, experimentally, with trien, had become intolerably allergic to the lifesaving drug penicillamine.

At about this same time, in the late 1970s and early 1980s:

A young woman with multiple sclerosis discovered that her hospitalization for treatment with the corticosteroid ACTH would not be reimbursed by her insurance carrier because the drug's manufacturers had never sought Food and Drug Administration (FDA) approval for that use.

The Centers for Disease Control (CDC) was running alarmingly short of the drug pentamidine for treating a heretofore rare type of pneumonia that had recently afflicted hundreds of immunosuppressed transplantation patients and was currently plaguing patients with AIDS (acquired immune deficiency syndrome).

A public health nurse in Kenya received a shipment of pneumococcal vaccine, days late and rendered potentially ineffective because a transportation breakdown had caused a lapse in refrigeration.

The National Cancer Institute (NCI) was continuing its massive program to identify and develop promising anticancer agents.

Several leading U.S. drug firms were making more than twenty experimental drugs available to clinical researchers to determine whether the drugs held any promise in treating patients with certain rare disorders.

And, a group of patients who had participated in clinical trials of an experimental drug for Parkinsons disease were afraid they would no longer be able to afford daily doses of the drug, now that it had been approved for marketing.

These dissimilar episodes have a common theme: They all involve *orphan drugs.* These are, simply stated, drugs that are medically important but are judged, on the basis of a host of market and regulatory factors, to be unprofitable by the pharmaceutical industry.

Orphan drugs are market losers because of the changing processes by which new drugs are discovered, developed, approved, and distributed in this country. They are, in essence, casualties of a system in flux. The changes in question pertain largely to the 1962 amendments to the Food, Drug and Cosmetic Act, which instituted the means to protect consumers from unsafe and ineffective drugs. As a result of these measures, however, a new drug now costs an estimated $50 million, on average, to develop and bring to the market. As a consequence, drugs with a low anticipated return on investment often do not undergo development as fast as technology would permit. Moreover, disincentives sidetrack orphan drugs at virtually every phase of the development cycle.

A brief description of this development process shows how plans can go awry. First, a chemical entity is screened for biologic activity or is synthesized using a known sequence; this is the *discovery* phase. Certain of these agents then are tested in animals to estimate their potential toxicity.

If the drug survives these preliminaries and if the sponsor decides to pursue human investigation, an application seeking approval for human clinical trials is submitted to the FDA; this application contains data on the method of drug production, and on the drug's quality, stability, toxicology, and pharmacology. If the drug is patentable, the sponsor takes out a patent on the drug either before or at the time the application for human testing is filed with the FDA.

Following approval of this application, the drug is given first to healthy volunteers to assess its safety in humans; then the drug is tested in a small number of patients to assess both safety and effectiveness. Finally, these properties, as well as optimum dose determinations, are tested in a larger number of patients.

Thereafter, the drug sponsor may apply to the FDA for approval to market the drug for the diseases ("indications") for which it has been tested. The FDA either approves the drug application for marketing or requests additional data be submitted in support of the marketing application. If the drug is approved by the FDA, the sponsor makes it available by prescription as the sole source of the drug if it is patented. The sponsor also assumes liability risks for adverse effects.

Problems with orphan drugs can arise during any of these steps. For instance, during early testing in patients with a complicated disease, establishing drug efficacy may be especially difficult, may take additional time and money, and still may not satisfy FDA requirements.

If the drug is not patentable, the company may decide it is not worthwhile to invest substantial sums in development, only to have their product copied and sold at a lower price by competitors that have not incurred any of the expense of developing the drug.

If the drug is highly toxic (as with anticancer drugs) or potentially toxic in some patients if taken over a long period of time (as with drugs for chronic disease), sponsors may be reluctant to take on added liability responsibility.

If the drug is approved for a common disease and later found effective in treating a rare disease, sponsors may decide it is not worth the expense to test and seek approval of the drug for use in this rare indication, since physicians legally can prescribe a drug for any indication once it is on the market. However, this practice means that the optimum dose may not have been worked out, that the drug is not reimbursable by health insurers, that possible multiple-drug interactions may not have been studied, and that the physician may be in an ambiguous liability situation if serious side effects do occur.

All these situations are greatly exacerbated if the drug is intended for a rare disease, which in commercial terms signifies a small market. Even if the sponsor decides to undertake premarket testing of a drug for a rare disease, it can be extremely difficult to find enough patients to participate in controlled clinical trials. This can result in long delays in completing premarket testing, and the developer still runs the risk of having insufficient data to establish efficacy.

During the past decade, problems of orphan drugs increasingly began to attract attention from those in government, academia, voluntary health agencies, and the pharmaceutical industry. Several categories of orphan drugs came to be recognized, including:

1. Drugs for rare diseases (small markets).
2. Drugs for chronic diseases (requiring longer periods of costly premarket safety and efficacy testing, with the patent clock ticking).
3. Drugs for single administration (vaccines and diagnostic aids, both of which have small market potential and high liability risks).
4. Drugs for women of childbearing age and for children (posing potential liability risks for the patient and/or developing fetus).
5. Drugs that are not patentable (shelf chemicals, natural substances, drugs known to exist, drugs that already have been patented for other uses).
6. Drugs for treating drug abuse (creating problems of image and liability, and encountering potential reluctance from users).
7. Drugs needed in Third World or developing nations (nonpaying customers with problems distributing and administering drugs).

Initially, discussion of orphan drugs was confined primarily to the rarefied atmosphere of medical journals. But patients and their families, whose lives were everyday reminders of the lack of solutions, soon turned to the press to publicize their plight. In concert with clinical researchers such as Melvin Van Woert and others, they made their frustration known to members of Congress. Perhaps nothing catapulted their problems into the public consciousness more poignantly than an episode on orphan drugs on the television show "Quincy." Within two years, an orphan drug bill aimed specifically at drugs for rare diseases, introduced by Representative Henry Waxman (D-Calif.) and Senator Nancy L. Kassebaum (R-Kan.), was passed by Congress and signed into law.

At the same time, a flurry of other activities on orphan drugs began. For instance, the Pharmaceutical Manufacturer's Association (PMA) established a Commission on Drugs for Rare Diseases, the FDA established an Office of Orphan Product Development, the Department of Health and Human Services (DHHS) set up an Orphan Products Board, and several of the voluntary health agencies banded together to form conjointly the National Organization for Rare Disorders (NORD).

Some economists have viewed the orphan drug problem as simply one of supply and demand. Some financial experts have viewed it as simply one of risk assessment. Some ethicists see it as a moral problem, and some scientists view it as basically a technological one. This book considers orphan drugs as a social problem, with economic, financial, ethical, and technological components.

The book looks at where the United States now stands with regard to orphan drugs. First, it examines the root problems that gave definition to the orphan drug profile and traces the interconnected changes in the drug development and regulatory processes that served to price certain drugs out of the market. Several aspects of the current situation are put into this perspective. Characteristics are discussed of known orphan drugs identified by their sponsors (both in the pharmaceutical industry and in government agencies) and surveyed by the Waxman Subcommittee on Health and the Environment, House Committee on Energy and Commerce. Thereafter, the strengths and weaknesses of recent legislation, and current government and industry responses are examined. Finally, some difficult residual questions are posed, including: Should drugs be developed for diseases no matter what the cost? If so, who should bear the economic burden? If not, on what basis should drug decisions be made? Finally, have we learned anything from the orphan drug experience that can be useful in addressing some of the other major issues affecting public-private sector interaction in the health care arena today?

John Walshe, the Cambridge University Wilsons disease specialist, summed up the orphan drug dilemma when he determined that this do-it-yourself drug development routine had gone on long enough and now should be placed on a sound commercial basis. This book attempts to assess how far, and how well, we have come in meeting that challenge.

2
A System in Change

L ouis Lasagna, professor of pharmacology and toxicology and medicine at the University of Rochester called the question in the journal *Regulation* in 1979, when he asked: who will adopt the orphan drugs?[1] In Lasagna's view, the problem needed flexible and imaginative solutions—adjectives he seldom applied to either industry or government. At a time, he continued, when technological innovation was poised for new advances, which were likely to be far different from those which produced the drugs of earlier decades, current costs of conforming to regulatory requirements were leaving promising but unprofitable drugs abandoned, and relegating certain groups of patients to therapeutic orphanhood.

How did this situation come about? A historical view suggests that even in the pharmaceutical industry's heyday in the 1950s, firms were reluctant to develop drugs that held little promise for profit. The federally funded anticancer drug development program was an example of industry's relative lack of interest. But the historical view also attributes industry reluctance to more stringent regulatory requirements that caused drug development costs to escalate and investment returns on drugs for rare diseases to plummet. In addition, the rising frequency and amount of liability awards further diminished enthusiasm for developing drugs for certain "orphan" populations, such as pregnant women, children, and mentally disabled patients.

Examining the evolving interrelationship between the pharmaceutical industry and its regulator, the Food and Drug Administration (FDA), permits orphan drug issues to be more appropriately placed into a larger context of drug development, approval, and distribution. Orphan drugs can be seen as a failure of a costly but otherwise socially desirable system to develop and distribute safe and effective medical drugs to those who need them. Protection against unsafe and ineffective drugs—which the public demands of its drug regulator, the FDA—has its costs. For instance, it has caused research and development (R&D) costs for establishing drug safety and efficacy to soar. As a result, development of certain medically important drugs that are not anticipated to recover their costs in the marketplace has slowed, if not halted.

Drug developers and regulators have responded to one another's actions, the developers through technical advances and breakthroughs and the regulators through legislation prompted by drug accidents and catastrophes. The result has been industrial competition based on drug R&D in an effort to find new market leaders, rather than on drug pricing. This is the crux of the issue for development of drugs for rare disorders.

This chapter describes the regulatory-industrial chain of events producing the current orphan status of many drugs; while the next chapter describes the increasing federal role as drug developer and liability insurer, and chapter 4 looks at the major technological breakthroughs that have transformed the nature of drug development, and at the implications of these changes for orphan drugs.

The Early Days of Drug Development

As Lewis Thomas, the *New England Journal of Medicine's* "biology watcher," relates in his recent autobiographical work, morphine was the only indispensable drug for his father, a physician practicing at the turn of the century.[2] Digitalis was next in value. In those days there was little a physician could do to change the course of a patient's illness. Nonetheless, wrote Thomas, his father filled out numerous prescriptions for each of his patients; placebos were the mainstay of medicine.

Indeed, according to medical historian James Harvey Young, few events served to distinguish drugs available in the early 1900s from those used 300 years earlier.[3] Until the late 1500s, drugs consisted of *galenicals* (usually plant extracts patterned after the ideas of Galen, the Greek physician of the second century A.D., who held that diseases resulted from an imbalance of the four humors—blood, phlegm, choler, and melancholy). By the late 1500s, chemicals, primarily minerals, had been added. By the mid-1600s the idea of patenting medicines took hold in Europe, and in the eighteenth century thousands of products were tested and endorsed, according to Silverman and Lee.[4] Although only two or three dozen of these were actually effective, the authors comment, many were memorable, including arsenic and marijuana.

English medical imports dominated the American market well into the early 1800s. During this period, however, the precursors of the modern pharmaceutical industry emerged in this country. Two major events facilitated the evolution of modern firms: passage of the Patent Act of 1790, which established market protection for certain medicines, and a technological breakthrough—the isolation of pure morphine from crude opium by a German physicist in 1805. This achievement later led to isolation of a number of other products, including quinine, codeine, atrophine, and cocaine, as well as naturally occurring vitamins and hormones.[5] Patent protection and technological innovation have both remained vital to the drug industry's strength, and the extent to which they both apply to a single product remains a central factor in drug development decisions.

The First Patents

The 1790 Patent Act set the period of protection at fourteen years, apparently because this was equivalent to two periods of apprenticeship. An 1836 act permitted the Commissioner of Patents to extend this term by an additional seven years, but this extension was repealed in the Patent Act of 1861 which established the current seventeen-year patent term. This appears to be a compromise between a House amendment granting an additional seven-year patent extension (to 21 years), and a Senate amendment favoring the fourteen-year limit. The law established several general principles: that a patentable invention must be a process, machine, manufacture, or composition of matter that is useful; that the invention must be novel and not obvious; and that an owner has the right to exclude others from making, using, or selling the invention in the United States. If the invention is made or used by or for the U.S. Government, however, the pantentee, though unable to prevent this infringement, can seek reasonable compensation.[6]

The patent specification provides information on how the invention is made, its utility, its uses, and the best modes of applying it. Finally, the specification provides claims defining the boundary of patent rights. Claims can cover a product (*product patent*), a process for product development (*process patent*), or a method for using the patent (*use patent*). Because the latter two forms are more difficult to enforce, the product patent remains the most important form of protection.

The Patent Act ushered in the means for industrial competition. Manufacturers of packaged medicines patented not only the medicines but also their method of composition and the distinctive shape of their containers, which did more than advertising to identify the medicines within. Manufacturers also secured twenty-eight-year copyrights on drug labels, renewable for an additional fourteen years, and began using the trademark. The emphasis on protecting the "look" of medicines was considered vital, since all drugs except narcotics were available over the counter. Consumers made purchase decisions, so marketing was aimed directly at them. The current practice of obtaining medicines by prescription is a relatively recent phenomenon, dating back only to the late 1930s, when the law governing food and drugs was amended. Patents were important during these early days of the industry, but it was not until technology paved the way for major new drug development in the mid-1930s that patents became an integral part of development decisions.

The Early Firms

The first holder of a U.S. patent for medicine (actually a device) in the late 1790s was a physician, Samuel Lee, who initiated the era of physician as medicine maker. A few small ventures ensued, originated by physicians seeking to make particular drugs easily available to their patients. Industry giants such as Upjohn, Abbott, and Eli Lilly trace their history back to these humble beginnings.

Meanwhile, chemical firms (engaged in making dyestuffs, fertilizers, and explosives) began producing drugs. Examples include Merck, Ciba-Geigy, and Pfizer. Bristol began as a bulk medicine supplier; several antibiotic producers, such as Schenley Laboratories (later of Riker Laboratories) developed from an interest in the fermentation process, whereas Smith Kline and French (now SmithKline Beckman) and McKesson and Barnes-Hind grew out of wholesale drug distribution firms. According to Silverman and Lee, Armour and others originated from the meat-packing industry, a source of hormones and other animal products.[7]

Early Regulations: 1906

These early firms lagged substantially behind European—especially German—companies in their U.S. market share, primarily as a result of technological rather than regulatory limitations. In fact, passage of the 1906 Pure Food and Drug Act did little to affect the pharmaceutical industry. Rather, the conditions of food production, processing, and packaging were the primary focus of the 1906 law, which was prompted in part by Upton Sinclair's account of conditions in the meat-packing industry described in his book *The Jungle*.[8]

The only provision concerning drugs in the 1906 law dealt solely with labels. They were to provide accurate descriptions of the drug's effects. Moreover, claims of infringement required proof of fraudulent intent in advertising.

In the early 1900s, U.S. firms continued to rely on European technology. But its entry into World War I forced the United States to close the technology gap. British, French, and U.S. firms turned their efforts to duplicating products previously available only from German firms. It was during this war period that U.S. firms began to gain a competitive advantage. As Massachusetts Institute of Technology (MIT) professor Peter Temin points out, technology was fixed. There was no need for research. Moreover, since the 1906 law did not change the way medicines were bought, advertising continued to be aimed at consumers. Therefore, competition between firms was based on drug price, and demand tended to be fairly elastic since consumers were price-conscious.[9]

It is easy to see why Lewis Thomas's father, as a general practitioner during this time, had so few therapeutic arrows in his sling. Medical education of the day emphasized only diagnosis and prognosis—the latter based on knowledge of the natural history of the disease in question. As Thomas concluded, this was the extent of science in medicine. Therapeutics were an empirical afterthought.[10]

The Modern Technological Era: 1932

For most historians, the year 1932, which saw the development of sulfanilamide, is credited as the beginning of the modern era of pharmaceuticals. At that time Lewis Thomas was completing his fourth year of medical school at Harvard. By then, Thomas reflects, medicine was becoming a technology based on "genuine science." Syphilis could be treated in its early stages by arsphenamine, although this was a difficult and hazardous therapy. Rabbit antipneumonococcal sera were being used to treat the most common forms of lobar pneumonia. Pernicious anemia was spectacularly reversed by liver extract (later attributed to the vitamin B12 in the extracts). Two elements of diabetes mellitus (elevated blood sugar and acidosis, which previously had led to coma and death) could be treated with the insulin preparation isolated by Banting and Best. Pellagra could be cured as a consequence of Goldberger's discovery of the vitamin B complex and identification of nicotinic acid. Finally, diphtheria could be prevented by immunization or treated with diphtheria antitoxin.[11]

Beyond all these advances, protonsil, developed in 1932 and introduced in 1935, stood out as a lifesaver in the treatment of infections. French scientists at the Pasteur Institute discovered that one element of the protonsil molecule consisted of sulfanilamide, a powerful antibacterial ingredient. Sulfanilamide's patent had long expired, since another of the molecule's components was a reddish dye that had been used for years as a dye-intermediate. Following widespread publicity in medical journals and newspapers worldwide, British, U.S., French, and German firms rushed to the market a number of sulfanilamide derivatives that could be patented.[12]

Prior to the introduction of sulfanilamide, only bed rest and nursing care could be offered for most infectious diseases. The most prevalent and fearsome of these were tuberculosis, tertiary syphilis, and rheumatic fever. With the dramatic news of sulfanilamide's potency, Thomas and his colleagues began to witness a profound change in the practice of medicine. When the first cases of pneumococcal and streptococcal septicemia were treated in Boston in 1937, Thomas recalls, a whole new world in medicine opened up. The profession had changed at the very moment of his entry.[13]

Regulatory Changes: 1938

With this technological explosion came a host of regulatory and legal changes in the form of new drug safety laws and new patent decisions. All these interacted to change the nature of the drug industry and the way industrial firms competed with one another.

The new wonder drug, sulfanilamide, was primarily responsible for new regulations on drug safety. According to Silverman and Lee, the Tennessee firm of Massengill & Co. sought to prepare a liquid form of the drug because, in its powder form, precise dosage was difficult to measure, and the drug had a bad taste. Sulfanilamide was found to dissolve in diethylene glycol, and it was sold as Elixir Sulfanilamide. According to the authors, however, it cannot be determined that the elixir was ever tested for safety in animals or humans. Such testing was not required by law. Shortly after the elixir was marketed, an American Medical Association (AMA) official received reports of possible drug-related deaths. He learned from the company that diethylene glycol had been the vehicle for sulfanilamide. Diethylene glycol was known to turn to fatal kidney-destroying oxalic acid in the body.[14] In total, the drug was blamed for the death of 100 people, most of them were children.[15] One victim was the chemist who had devised the elixir; he committed suicide.

In the few years preceding this tragedy, the Department of Agriculture (of which FDA was then a constituent agency) had been mounting an ambitious effort to rewrite its basic statutory authority. The department had sought to widen its powers over drug regulation and to circumvent cumbersome court procedures it had to follow to remove a drug from the market. Congress, busy with what were considered far more pressing economic reforms of the Depression era, gave little attention to the department's efforts.

In 1935, a bill drawn up by New Deal brain trust member Rexford Guy Tugwell, undersecretary of agriculture, passed the House but not the Senate. The following year, 1936, a Senate bill passed, but differences between the House and Senate versions were not resolved by the end of the session and the bill died. A new bill was introduced in 1937 and again passed the heavily Democratic house but ran into bitter opposition in the more conservative Senate. There was intense lobbying against it by the food, drug, and cosmetic industries, the last of these about to be brought under federal regulation for the first time under this measure.

It was in this congressional atmosphere that the sulfanilamide disaster dissolved opposition to the Food, Drug and Cosmetic Act of 1938, which was rushed through Congress. It empowered the FDA to strengthen the labeling requirements by assuring that appropriate warnings had been included, banned excessively dangerous drugs from the market, and strengthened enforcement procedures. Most important from a safety standpoint, it required manufacturers to submit to FDA evidence that the drug was relatively safe.[16] Nonetheless, the burden was on the FDA to demonstrate that a drug was *not* safe in order to keep it off the market. FDA had a fixed period of time within which to approve a drug application; if FDA's safety review had not been completed within that period, or had not been extended by new data requests, the drug automatically became marketable. Once marketed under these procedures, a drug was almost immune to FDA challenge in the absence of overwhelming legal proof of its dangers.

Although the new labeling clause under the act did not receive as much attention as the safety provisions, it also had a major impact. As Peter Temin from MIT notes in his interesting article on the nature of competition in the drug industry, regulations resulting from FDA's interpretation of the labeling provisions created for the first time a distinction between over-the-counter and prescription drugs.[17] The former were to have detailed labels; the latter would have limited labels but would be available only through a physician's prescription. According to Temin, most drugs introduced after the 1938 law were prescription drugs. Drug advertising underwent an immediate metamorphosis: Its focus shifted toward physicians rather than price-conscious consumers. Thereafter, drug prices began to reflect the new state of inelastic demand, since prescribers rather than payers were making drug choice decisions. Moreover, changes soon to come in the patent law interpretation solidified the state of inelastic demand following the discovery and introduction of the next two wonder drugs, penicillin and streptomycin.

Patent Interpretation Changes: The 1940s

In the mid-1940s, shortly after sulfanilamide became available, penicillin was developed as a therapeutic agent. Not without difficulty, however: According to an account by Richard Harris, penicillin—produced from common mold and initially found effective against bacteria—also was found by two British scientists in 1941 to be efficacious in treating septic wounds. U.S. officials were anxious to see if it could be produced in quantity to treat battlefield wounds. Vannevar Bush, director of the U.S. Office of Scientific Research and Development, induced several companies to work on the problem. But concerns over protection of patent claims on the methods of production precluded exchange of information by the firms involved. Eventually, Department of Agriculture scientists at the Peoria, Illinois, lab developed a large-scale production method, filed a departmental patent application, and made the patent available to any producer without charge. Stiff pricing competition among manufacturers soon drove the cost down from $200 to 60 cents per million units.[18]

Next came streptomycin, the first new antibiotic since penicillin. The events surrounding its development and marketing brought a triumviral transformation of the drug industry, involving changes in technology, patent rights, and organizational structure, which together shaped the industry of today, as the following discussion adapted in large part from Temin's article, shows.

Technological and Legal Changes

The transformation began in the 1940s, when Selman Waksman at Rutgers University discovered a technique for screening soil samples to find new antibiotics, based on methods used to discover penicillin. He hypothesized that since harmful microorganisms did not survive in the ground, soil probably contained substances that killed them. Streptomycin was soon discovered, demonstrating that penicillin was not a unique phenomenon but, rather, the first in a series of important new drugs, which, through this screening technique, lay within scientific reach.

The discovery of streptomycin precipitated another major change concerning patents. The Patent and Trademark Office ruled that, although streptomycin was a natural substance and therefore not patentable as such, its natural form was not useful medically. Although streptomycin was developed from a natural mold, it was a transitory product of nature that had not been isolated previously. Moreover, its therapeutic use had not been known. The office therefore ruled that both the chemical modifications that permitted purification and the new product itself were patentable. This interpretation signified that all future antibiotics also could be considered patentable. Despite this bonanza, streptomycin's manufacturer, Merck, did not reap the extra benefits. Instead, Waksman convinced Merck to make production available through an unrestricted license, according to Temin, on the basis that public (that is, university) facilities had been used for an important public health discovery and therefore should not be so used for private gain.

Merck agreed. It assigned its patents to the Rutgers Research Foundation; used the patent; and sold streptomycin under its generic form, in competition with other companies, to independent packagers and distributors. As with penicillin, competition soon forced streptomycin's price down during the 1950s, but Waksman's generous concept, agreed to by Merck, did not take hold. With few exceptions, the practice of making a patent available to other manufacturers came to an abrupt halt, except in instances of using restricted licenses, which will be discussed.

The idea that universities should seek patent rights for pharmaceuticals was then quite new because chemistry was the basis of pharmacology, and pharmacological chemists generally worked for pharmaceutical firms rather than at universities. As will be discussed later, this situation has changed dramatically in the past decade as new molecular biology techniques, developed at universities, have occasioned a myriad of new industry-university arrangements in which patent rights play a central role.

After the development of streptomycin, patents became an integral component of competition. They, along with a new emphasis on advertising, precipitated the third major aspect of the industrial transformation: vertical integration of firms. This organizational change, in concert with the technological and legal ones, completed the triangular new foundation of the industry.

Organizational Changes: Vertical Integration

Heretofore, drug firms were primarily manufacturers which relied on packagers and distributors to market their products. Now, however, as Peter Temin shows, new technological possibilities and liberal patent right interpretations prompted firms to become innovators as well as manufacturers. Unrestricted product licensing gave way to the use of patent rights and the retention of a monopoly over new drug production. This production of drugs was geared to maximizing profits by restricting output: Only the amount that could be sold at the high market price would be produced.

With the practice of retaining patents, firms became vertically integrated, incorporating innovation, manufacturing, packaging, distributing, and marketing functions for their drugs as a means to control these. Temin notes that firms could have decided to license other producers and command a royalty payment of 80 percent of sales; this would have kept market prices similarly high. He suggests that the exclusive-production approach already was set in place in other industries, and that exclusive production meshed better with advertising plans. *Detail men* (company representatives who visit physicians and provide information on a company's products) were becoming an important marketing vehicle now that most medicines were obtained by doctors' prescriptions; these men could represent an exclusively marketed product better than one that was widely licensed.

During these first years of vertical integration, competition for market share for a single drug was also changing. The broad-spectrum antibiotics that followed the discovery and introduction of streptomycin were prime examples of the new major change from nonexclusive licensing to restricted production, according to Temin. But the similarity of the next three broad-spectrum drugs (chlortetracycline, chloramphenicol, and oxytetracycline) caused competition among them to increase, which in turn caused the price to fall. Although patent monopoly and marketing organization were necessary for the creation of market power, they were not sufficient. At this point, companies turned to research for help.[19]

Emergence of Research-Intensive Firms

By this time, in the mid- to late 1940s, the great drug-therapy era that had begun with the introduction of sulfanilamide, penicillin, and streptomycin had produced the means for slashing the death rates from rheumatic fever, childbed fever, and pneumonia. Drugs could save lives threatened by scarlet fever, meningococcal meningitis, staphylococcal infection, and typhoid fever.[20] Moreover, syphilis—which Lewis Thomas and his colleagues in their early days of training had treated apprehensively with arsphenamine—now could be dramatically treated, safely and effectively, with penicillin. Malaria, contracted in the tropics, responded to treatment with quinine derivatives and other antimalarials.

The competing broad-spectrum antibiotics were essentially patentable "me too" drugs developed by three newly integrated firms: Lederle (chlortetracycline), Parke-Davis (chloramphenicol), and Pfizer (oxytetracycline). In an attempt to improve its competitive advantage in a sagging market, newcomer Pfizer developed a new drug, tetracycline, through a modification of the chemical structure of Lederle's drug. As Temin relates, Parke-Davis reactivated its research in this area, and two additional firms, Bristol and Hayden Chemical Corporation, found they had made tetracycline using a different method. The legal position was intricate. According to Temin, however, the firms settled the dispute among themselves rather than allowing the Patent Office to make a ruling. By means of acquisitions, private agreements, and licensing arrangements, the five firms ended up marketing tetracycline under Pfizer's product patent and thereby arresting the price decline. In what came to be termed the *antibiotic cartel*, the firms determined the market price for the drugs—one that would remain constant for a decade.[21]

A similar situation occurred with cortisone. As Richard Harris describes in his book on the amendments, cortisone was first developed at the Mayo Clinic by Eric Kendall in 1936. Isolated from extracts from animal adrenal cortex, its scarcity made it difficult to secure enough material to conduct clinical tests. After some years of effort, Lewis Sarett of Merck discovered a way to synthesize cortisone from ox bile. In 1948, clinical studies with cortisone were conducted at the Mayo Clinic. From the initial work it appeared that the hormone might be beneficial in a number of conditions, including rheumatoid arthritis, intractable asthma, lupus, gout, Addisons disease, Hodgkins disease, lymphatic leukemia, rheumatic fever, and tetanus. Initially the hormone had cost $4,800 per ounce (more than 100 times the price of gold), as Harris points out. Merck scientists had cut down on the thirty-seven steps required to produce it. Then in 1952, scientists at Upjohn devised a method of producing the hormone by fermentation of Mexican yams. This further reduced the necessary steps. However, the therapeutic effects were short-lived, the hormone proved congenial to microorganisms, and the drug had acute side effects.

In 1955, Schering Corporation marketed two new adrenocortical steroids, prednisone and prednisolone. These were more potent than cortisone, appeared to demonstrate fewer side effects, and were considered by the Patent and Trademark Office to be a significant enough improvement on nature to be patentable. Schering, Upjohn, Merck, Pfizer, and Parke-Davis all applied for patents. The firms agreed that the company that won the patent award would license the drug on a royalty basis to the other companies with patent claims. No additional firms would be able to buy the material in bulk (that is, in powder form, needing only to be put into tablets and packaged). Enter Syntex—a small company at the time—which independently marketed the drug, asserting, according to Harris, that it actually had discovered prednisone first. Syntex manufactured bulk prednisone, sold it to small companies, and eventually made customers of Merck and Pfizer.[22] With the following generation of synthetic steroids and contraceptive pills, however, exclusive production became the order of the day in the hormone product category too. According to Temin, the companies involved grew rapidly, as had those marketing broad-spectrum antibiotics.

In Temin's view, these technological innovations led to patent monopolies which were exercised as monopoly production rather than through restricted licensing. The ensuing competition among manufacturers of similar patented products prompted vertical integration of firms. This resulted in greater profits, which in turn produced larger companies. Drug industry profits, which had been high relative to total manufacturing profits in general before introduction of these new technologies, remained similarly high afterward. But the new technologies did not enable the drug industry to further widen the gap between its profits and those of other manufacturers. Rather, the leading firms then increased their advertising and R&D expenditures as their primary means of competition, rather than competing by lowering drug prices. These expenditures reduced profits, though not to the competitive level. Patents conferred temporary market power on discoverers of new drugs, but patent monopolies (unlike, for instance, Eastman's patent monopoly in photography) did not create a single dominant firm. The new technology involved methods of research rather than production, and hence could not be patented. Competition among drugs for similar uses offset the market power of patents over time. Therefore, Temin concludes that it is difficult to determine whether these technological and regulatory changes increased market power in the industry. The lack of price competition and the resultant maintenance of high drug prices suggest they did. But, he adds, the apparent failure of high drug industry profits to rise even higher relative to general manufacturing profits suggests they did not.[23]

The major implication of Temin's analysis for orphan drugs is that competition in the 1950s was inefficient. It did not lower prices for drugs protected by patent but, rather, caused costs to rise to approach those prices. To the extent that these added costs were incurred to capture market share, rather than to develop socially useful products or better inform consumers, the competition had no social product.

This analysis suggests that even in the 1950s, during the boom in new drug introductions, drugs with small markets and those that were not patentable were unlikely candidates for inclusion in the industry's competitive strategy. Although unpatentable drugs and those for rare diseases were not major beneficiaries of these industrial shifts, other drugs were and represented major therapeutic advances, including some which were molecular modifications of existing drugs. Among these, as Temin points out, were: erythromycin, a powerful new broad-spectrum antiobiotic (Lilly and Abbott); chlorothiazide, a thiazide diuretic derived from the sulfa drugs (Merck, Sharp and Dohme); tolbutamide (Upjohn) and chlorpropamide (Pfizer), oral hypoglycemics for diabetes which were derived from the sulfonamides; cortisone (Syntex, Upjohn and others); reserpine, the sedative and anti-hypertensive (Ciba); and chlorpromazine, a major tranquilizer (Smith Kline and French, now SmithKline Beckman). Moreover, these drugs became major sources of revenue for their firms in the 1950s. In fact, as Temin and Schwartzman both conclude, firms were reliant on one or two drugs for most of their profits; remaining products generally did little more than cover costs.[24] A recent report issued by the U.S. Congress Office of Technology Assessment (OTA) on Patent-Term Extension suggests that this situation persists today.[25]

The shift in competition away from drug prices and toward research on patentable large-market drugs, and more efficient and effective advertising to physicians, were major factors in stimulating interest in the drug industry by the Senate Antitrust and Monopoly Subcommittee in the late 1950s. According to Harris's account, a Schering official summed up the situation during hearings in an exchange with Senator Estes Kefauver (D-Tenn.), the subcommittee chairman. The Schering official, when asked why companies don't lower their prices if they actually want to be competitive, responded that you can't count two people for every one person who is sick. A Premo official acknowledged that the only real competition in the industry was for the physician's attention through advertising.[26]

Thus although some industry sources have suggested that orphan drugs essentially resulted from the next major legislative change— namely, the 1962 Kefauver-Harris amendments to the Food, Drug and Cosmetic Act—Temin's analysis suggests that the origins of the problem could be found in the industry's organizational structure and marketing strategy of the late 1950s.

The year 1955 had been the peak for introduction of new drug applications, with 357 approved, according to Donald Kennedy, a former FDA commissioner and currently president of Stanford University.[27] Thereafter there was a steady decline in new applications, a trend that has continued to some extent to the present, and one that was greatly intensified after the 1962 amendments to the Food, Drug and Cosmetic Act. As the OTA Patent-Term Extension report indicates, however, the number of new chemical entities (NCEs) approved by the FDA has remained relatively constant since 1963, as has the number of NCEs (as assessed by FDA) offering important therapeutic gain.[28] But even as the number of new drug applications was just beginning its descent, none of the drugs in the 1955–1959 period were *public service* drugs (an industry term for *orphan* drugs) intended for narrow use, as noted by Barry Bloom, vice-president of research for Pfizer, Inc.[29]

The National Cancer Institute (NCI) probably was the first federal research agency to recognize the problems involved in developing drugs for rare diseases. That institute, in the same year the number of new drug applications peaked (1955), embarked on a federal anticancer drug program which was to become a major contributor to every facet of cancer drug therapy from that time on. NCI's program presented clear evidence that drugs for at least some small markets were already conspicuously absent from the development plans of drug companies by the late 1950s. Nevertheless, a list compiled in 1965 by the Pharmaceutical Manufacturer's Association (PMA) indicates that industry was providing thirty-eight service drugs. Most of these were in experimental stages (a few were for laboratory use only); but at least four of the drugs were commercially available, some without charge. These drugs ranged from poison antidotes to diagnostic dyes, antidepressants, a few for certain forms of carcinoma, and others. Nevertheless no one disputes that the problem of

orphan drugs, if indeed it existed in the 1950s, was greatly exacerbated after the 1962 Kefauver-Harris amendments to the 1938 Food,
Drug and Cosmetic Act.

The 1962 Amendments

The 1962 Kefauver-Harris amendments to the Food, Drug and Cosmetic Act restructured the way drugs are approved in this country.
This in turn affected the way drugs are developed, and may have
also affected decisions determining which drugs to develop. The 1962
amendments were the next major event to shape the evolution of
the regulatory-industrial transformation begun in the 1930s.

Just as the sulfanilamide tragedy precipitated the 1938 law, so
the thalidomide disaster of 1962 precipitated the 1962 amendments.
Thalidomide had resulted in terrible birth deformities in infants born
to mothers who, during pregnancy, were prescribed the apparently
safe tranquilizer by European doctors. The thalidomide tragedy gal-
vinized Senator Estes Kefauver's efforts to introduce entirely new
safety and efficacy requirements into the regulatory process. Kefauver's antitrust bill, initially based on his effort to promote increased
industrial competition and thereby lower drug prices, eventually was
rewritten along the lines originally proposed by Representative Leo-
nor K. Sullivan (D-Mo.). Through her 1961 bill (H.R. 1235), she was
the first member of Congress to propose efficacy requirements be
introduced into drug regulation, a stance later adapted by the Kennedy administration at the time Senator Kefauver's bill was undergoing final revision.

After the thalidomide disclosures, the Kefauver antitrust bill
eventually became law without any of its antitrust provisions. Instead, it covered aspects of drug safety and efficacy through provisions affecting drug testing and approval, labeling, advertising, and
monitoring of firms. The new regulations developed by FDA to implement the law have been credited with improving the safety and
establishing the efficacy standards for drug approval, and improving
access to information about side effects, but concurrently causing
drug development costs to skyrocket. All these factors have been
recognized as creating particularly acute problems for orphan drugs.

Background to the Amendments

Estes Kefauver, chairman of the Senate Subcommittee on Antitrust
and Monopoly, and his staff initially were concerned about drug

prices, which were considered high and noncompetitive. Much of the information about subcommittee deliberations comes from an account by Richard Harris, who followed the subcommittee's actions on the amendments. He relates that staff were astounded to learn that three brands of antibiotics (Chloromycetin, marketed by Parke-Davis; Aureomycin, marketed by Lederle; and Terramycin, marketed by Pfizer) all had exactly the same retail price. Similarly, the four largest companies selling prednisone and prednisolone (Schering, Merck, Upjohn, and Pfizer) all charged the same price for these drugs—a price that had not changed since their 1956 market introduction.[30] Aware of the patent dispute over these two drugs, staff reportedly were concerned that the companies preferred to decide by private agreement who should retain patent rights rather than settle by litigation.

Additionally, staff wanted to explore the possibility that the industry was using administered-price techniques, a concept that, as analyzed by the noted New Deal economist Gardiner Means, concluded that prices were being administered when demand decreases were matched by production decreases in order to keep prices at the same level. This analysis fits with that later suggested by Temin, who noted that industry obtained monopoly profits by restricting output. Means proposed that signs of administered prices could be seen when companies with different cost and profit profiles sold a product at the same price, and when large companies followed the pricing lead of the largest company. Added interest in the situation occurred when Kefauver's colleague, Senator Warren Magnuson (D-Wash.), found that some U.S.-made drugs were selling in Sweden at only 20 percent of their U.S. retail cost.

According to Harris, subcommittee staff learned from Federal Trade Commission (FTC) reports that drug industry profits of 18.9 percent of invested capital after taxes and 10.8 percent of sales after taxes were twice as high as the average for all manufacturing entities listed in the report.[31] Fueled by these facts and figures, the subcommittee embarked on a series of hearings from 1958 to 1961 concerning competition in the drug industry. Their main problem was lack of information on production costs; without it, they had little on which to base a thorough price investigation. This obstacle was pushed aside when the staff learned from industry-submitted documents that the margin between basic production costs and selling price could be determined. According to Harris, staff discovered that Schering purchased prednisolone from Upjohn for $2.37 per gram. They then calculated that a 5 milligram tablet of Meticortelone cost Schering slightly more than 1 cent. The druggist paid 18 cents, and the consumer paid 30 cents. The $2.37/gram figure included Upjohn's profit, so the 1 cent per tablet figure was conservative. When staff then added in the costs of tableting, the total production cost came to 1.567 cents per tablet, including profit to both the actual producer (Upjohn) and the firm tableting and bottling the material, according to Harris. After this information was presented at the hearings, newspapers reported that a drug costing 1.57 cents sold for 17.9 cents— a markup of 1,118 percent. Another drug (estradiol progynon, used to treat menopausal disorders) purchased by Schering from the French firm Roussel, was reported by subcommittee staff at that hearing to have a 7,079 percent markup, based on the same kind of calculations.[32] Although these headlines generated intense interest in the pricing of pharmaceuticals, legislative action on Kefauver's Antitrust proposals seemed unlikely.

Other issues were also defined during the hearings. John Lear, science editor of the *Saturday Review*, reported on concerns expressed by some academic physicians with whom he had consulted about "new" combination drugs. Under terms of the 1938 act, clearance was relatively easy for previously approved drugs which were combined and promoted as new drugs. There were dozens of such combination drugs on the market, most of which appeared to be no more efficacious than their component drugs used alone. This view was reiterated by Dr. Maxwell Finland, an infectious-disease specialist at Harvard Medical School, who said that hundreds of drug combinations were marketed that did not necessarily have therapeutic advantages over the same drugs taken separately. As a former medical officer at FDA pointed out at the hearing, no drug is safe if it fails to work while an effective drug is available. Also of concern was the fact that, since no drug is totally safe, ineffective drugs are therefore unnecessarily unsafe.

A Library of Congress study authorized by Kefauver looked at advertisements of thirty-four widely used trade-named drugs appearing in medical journals between July 1958 and March 1959. The study concluded that eighty-nine percent of ads contained either no mention or minimal mention of side effects. Although the current law stipulated that side effects were to be described in package inserts accompanying each shipment of new drugs approved by FDA, these inserts went to the pharmacist, not to the physician. Subcommittee staff questioned whether physicians had adequate and easy access to information on drug contraindications.[33]

Finally, Kefauver wanted to create a means for improving the competitive position of smaller ethical companies (those that produce prescription drugs) and of generic drug firms (those that manufacture and/or sell prescription drugs not protected by patent) with respect to the larger ethical drug companies. One possible solution was to ensure that the manufacturing practices of generic and small companies were as uniformly reliable as those of major manufacturing companies. This might make physicians more confident about prescribing less expensive versions of the same drug. Physicians considered this problem important from a liability standpoint since, although hospitals often had the facilities to test generic drugs for bioequivalency, individual physicians did not. Therefore, they were less likely to trust generics or drugs marketed by smaller companies.

Generic drugs, or bioequivalent versions of drugs that are unpatented, had been available throughout this period. Initially these drugs were manufactured by production-intensive companies. However, research-intensive companies began developing "branded" generic drugs as well as their trade-named drugs. Since generic drugs were produced by both research-intensive and production-intensive companies, both groups conceivably could benefit from measures seeking increased sales of unpatented drugs. However, brand-name generic drugs of research-intensive firms tended to fare better in the marketplace because they carried the firm's name and reputation. Thus subcommittee staff anticipated that these manufacturing-standards provisions would benefit production-intensive companies by reassuring physicians that the drugs were manufactured under conditions and by processes that FDA judged to meet the standard.

The hearings also revealed allegations that some top level FDA officials were more concerned about maintaining good relationships with industry than with supporting their own staff reviewers' decisions to ask firms for additional data. Representative Sullivan had put Senator Kefauver in touch with one former FDA pharmacologist, Barbara Moulton, who testified about this problem. Sitting in on the hearings was Frances Kelsey, a pharmacologist who was currently working at FDA. She would later, through stalling and finally preventing approval of thalidomide for sale in the United States, become a central figure in demonstrating the need for stricter safety regulations.

Dr. Moulton's testimony suggested that the FDA had been "captured" by the pharmaceutical industry. Capture theory suggests that members of regulatory agencies fall into step with the firms they regulate, particularly when there is a so-called revolving door between government and private employment. Capture theory has taken two basic forms. As summarized in the *Wharton Magazine*, the *natural life cycle school*, advocated by sociologists, legal scholars, and political scientists, views the formation of the regulatory agency as a response to public pressures, which recede once the agency is formed. The agency then strikes a bargain with the industry it regulates. Some agency personnel leave rather than be captured. The second or *economic school* is itself composed of two factions. One considers commissioners as acting in their own behalf or self-interest because their tenure is short-lived; they maintain good relations with industry in the knowledge that they are likely to enter industry or politics once they leave the regulatory agency. The second branch—the *purchase* approach—suggests that policymaking is purchased by the industry through political alliances with federal legislative and executive branch officials.[34] Leaving aside the issue of whether the FDA was considered either by internal or external groups to be captured by industry, Harris reports that Kefauver complained of getting little help from FDA during the course of the hearings. A House staff member familiar with the legislation, however, reported that FDA Commissioner George Larrick had been instrumental in identifying for Representative Sullivan a number of serious loopholes in the 1938 act dealing with safety provisions. Larrick also stressed the need for establishing an efficacy requirement. These suggestions were then covered in Representative Sullivan's bill and later in the Kefauver bill, according to staff member Charles Holstein.

Not until the horrifying effects of thalidomide devastated public consciousness about unsafe drugs did passage of a drug safety bill take on urgency. Infants of mothers using thalidomide during pregnancy were born with phocomelia, which meant they were missing all or part of their legs or arms. The drug, developed by the West German firm Chemie Grunenthal, was linked to phocomelia in children born in Sweden, Italy, Great Britain, Scotland, Switzerland, Lebanon, Israel, Australia, Brazil, and Peru as well as West Germany. Thalidomide, under the name Kevadon, was being licensed from Chemie Grunenthal by Merrell and marketed in Canada. FDA pharmacologist Frances Kelsey was credited with keeping the drug off the U.S. market by repeatedly requesting additional information from Merrell while quietly investigating the facts behind a report in the *British Medical Journal* suggesting that certain cases of peripheral neuritis might be related to thalidomide. According to Harris, Kelsey's concerns were prompted by her awareness from earlier research that drugs that irritated nerves in adult rabbits could stunt growth and produce deformity in the rabbit's fetus. By asking for more data, FDA could avoid having the drug enter the market if a safety determination had not been reached before the regulatory deadline period expired.

After later epidemiological evidence linked the drug with the deformities, Chemie Grunenthal withdrew all forms of the drug from distribution and sale in November 1961. Merrell withdrew its brand from the Canadian market three months later, according to Harris. But Merrell had sent the drug to more than 1,200 U.S. doctors for testing; estimates were that 20,000 patients had received the experimental drug. At the time, companies were required only to keep records of shipments of experimental drugs and to warn on the label that the drug was limited to investigational use. Physicians receiving investigational drugs were required only to sign a statement that they were qualified to test the drug. They were not required to inform patients that the drug was experimental.

FDA moved to warn those who had received the drug and those physicians who might be dispensing it. But the agency was unable to track down 99 of the more than 1,200 physicians provided with the drug. According to Harris, more than 400 physicians who had been alerted by FDA had not tried to contact their patients who received supplies of the drug. Reportedly, many of these physicians had not kept records of the drug's distribution. Some officials at FDA as well as subcommittee staff also suspected that many were afraid of liability repercussions.[35]

The situation highlighted serious gaps in the process of testing and tracking experimental drugs. Thalidomide had demonstrated obvious flaws in (1) controlling the dissemination of investigational drugs, (2) being certain that patients knew of the experimental nature of drugs they were taking, (3) having effective means of recalling doubtful or dangerous experimental drugs, and (4) assuring that participating physicians maintained adequate records on the effects of these drugs. There were other flaws as well. FDA officials stated that quite a few cases of falsified research data were on file, and suggested that these cases fell into two categories: Some physicians being paid to test new drugs either altered research data or performed no actual tests. Other physicians based their reports on a few uncontrolled trials. Moreover, there had been a few reported cases of drug companies themselves falsifying data submitted to FDA, as described by Silverman and Lee.[36]

Even before the Kefauver-Harris amendments passed, thalidomide caused the agency to issue new regulations covering drug testing. As announced by Anthony Celebrezze, secretary of the Department of Health, Education and Welfare (DHEW; now Department of Health and Human Services, DHHS), drug sponsors were to:

1. Inform FDA on the distribution of drugs for investigational use.

2. Use only qualified investigators whose qualifications were to be filed with the government.
3. Test no new drugs in humans until safety had been demonstrated in animals.
4. Inform FDA of the progress of human testing.
5. Take special precautions with drugs intended for use by pregnant women or by children.[37]

Thalidomide had mobilized the administration and the Congress as well. With the Kennedy White House staff placing new emphasis on prodding Congress to enact a strong drug bill—and after a series of complex negotiations between House and Senate committees, including input from White House and DHEW staff—a final version cleared the Congress and was signed into law in 1962.

In sum, the factors that had motivated the Kefauver subcommittee included: lack of demonstrated efficacy of existing and new drugs; minimal reporting to doctors and regulators of adverse effects of drugs and lack of effective means to track and recall dangerous experimental drugs; drug prices that were considered high and monopolistically noncompetitive by subcommittee standards; and lack of physician trust in generic products because there was no assurance of uniformity of manufacturing practices. The aims of the House-passed Harris bill, sponsored by Representative Orren Harris, (D-Ark.), chairman of the House Committee on Interstate and Foreign Commerce, were to assure consumers that drugs available on the market were safe and effective. As Richard Harris points out, Kefauver accomplished everything he wanted in the House-Senate conference bill—except his much-desired provisions to lower drug prices, which were the focus of his original measure before the thalidomide disaster prompted him to widen its scope. Although the antitrust features of Senator Kefauver's bill were properly in the jurisdiction of his Senate Judiciary Subcommittee, the drug safety and clearance provisions of the final bill were actually in the jurisdiction of another Senate committee, Labor and Education. That committee's chairman, Senator Lister Hill, who was a major force in health legislation, graciously stood aside to let his colleague from Tennessee preside over the amendments.

Features of the Amended Law

The amendments set new requirements for establishing drug safety and efficacy before drugs could be approved for marketing in interstate commerce. They also included measures for strengthening the competitive position of generic and small ethical drug companies, and set new criteria for information to be used in advertisements and labeling.

Specifically, the provisions of S. 1552 included, with regard to drug safety:

1. Abolition of the previous provision granting automatic approval of a new drug application after a fixed period of time.
2. Requirement that firms keep records on all reported adverse effects of drugs.
3. Certification by FDA of each batch of all antibiotics, at industry expense.

With respect to improving the potential competitive position of small firms and generic drug manufacturers, and also with regard to safety:

4. Strict factory inspections were to be conducted by FDA.
5. Improved standards of quality control in manufacturing were to be set up.

Specifically with regard to generic drug recognition:

6. All labels and all advertising and promotional materials were to have the drug's generic name in letters at least one-half the size of the drug's trade-name letters.
7. DHEW was to review all generic names and establish simpler ones where necessary.

Toward improving information available on drugs:

8. FDA was to reject new drug applications and withdraw approved drugs in cases of false drug labeling.
9. Package inserts were to be distributed with drugs going to all physicians, hospitals, and medical facilities.
10. All advertisements were to include information on the drug's efficacy and side effects.

Additionally:

11. The Patent and Trademark Office had the right to ask FDA about drugs on file with FDA.

12. The names and addresses of all pharmaceutical firms were to be listed with FDA.
13. All drugs were to be shown to have proof of efficacy, including not only those developed after the new amendments but also those already on the market.[38]

Although all the provisions of the 1962 amendments had a major impact on the industry and on FDA, the first group, concerning safety, and the last, concerning efficacy, have had the most profound effects on the development of all drugs—particularly with respect to orphan drugs.

New Procedures for Drug Approval

Following enactment of the amended law, all new applications to market a drug were required to show, through adequate tests, the drug's safety for use under conditions prescribed in the proposed drug label. Additionally, drug sponsors had to show substantial evidence of effectiveness in those uses through adequate, well-controlled studies. Finally, identity, strength, quality, and purity of the drug had to be established through information on the manufacture, quality control, and chemical process used, according to a Review Panel on New Drug Regulation.[39]

Although the 1938 law had called for review of drug safety information by FDA, a drug was automatically approved if FDA did not either rule against the safety data within a stipulated, fixed period of time, or request additional data. The 1962 amendments called for FDA to take positive action to approve a new drug application based on satisfaction that data showed safety and substantial evidence of effectiveness. Without this approval, the drug would not be allowed to be shipped in interstate commerce, although some distributors later avoided these restrictions by manufacturing and distributing unapproved drugs within an individual state.

Duration and scope of clinical and animal trials to evaluate safety and efficacy were to be a function of the drug's complexity, its therapeutic potential, its intended use, its novelty, and other factors.

The IND Process

Under a new process established by FDA for implementing the law, before any studies could commence in humans, the drug sponsor was required to submit to FDA a Notice of Claim for Investigational Exemption of a New Drug, referred to as an IND. Legally, the IND exempts the manufacturer of an experimental drug from the federal prohibition against shipping an unapproved drug product in interstate commerce. Operationally, it sets up a three-stage procedure for drug testing. The three stages are outlined prospectively in an investigational new drug (IND) application, provided by the drug sponsor to the FDA. The IND includes plans for testing the drug: first, in a small number of healthy volunteers, to assess safety; next, in a small number of patients, to assess safety and efficacy in treating the disease for which the drug is intended; and, finally, in a large number of patients, to assess safety, efficacy, and optimum dose. These three phases of clinical trials will be described in detail.

As Schwartzman explains, companies usually pursue new drug candidates in fields in which the company has made a commitment to establish expertise. The process of drug discovery leading to the IND plan has relied on generating a working hypothesis that seeks to explain the underlying nature of a disease and how this disease process may be arrested, prevented, or reversed by particular compounds. Choice of specific compounds likely to be effective is based in part on information about the pharmacologic action of drugs previously used to treat the disease. An important consideration at this point is whether there exists an appropriate animal model (or, lately, an equivalent such as a tissue culture model) of the human disease. Once candidate compounds are synthesized, scientists test compounds for biologic activity and determine which of them have the desired biologic effect with the least toxicity. As Schwartzman emphasizes, most of the drug discoveries of the past originated from naturally occurring compounds, accidental discoveries, or modifications of previously known drugs.

Compounds that survive the initial screening are entered into secondary screens for more extensive study; simultaneously, they undergo additional primary screens to determine whether they may have potential therapeutic effects in other fields or whether they have any additional adverse effects. Often, according to Schwartzman, these additional primary screens involve studying the drug's action on the cardiovascular, pulmonary, renal, and central nervous systems. Large companies are at an advantage here since their laboratories can support major research projects in a number of therapeutic fields. Patents may be taken out at this point or sometime during this period, but no later than the time at which preclinical data are submitted to FDA in the IND application.

According to Schwartzman, early animal tests can provide at best only inferences of safety and efficacy. Intensive animal toxicology and pharmacology tests are initiated to determine the high-low dose range (the highest dose that causes obvious side effects but does not kill the animal; the mid- or second dose range, which causes borderline side effects; and the low dose range, which is the maximum dose at which no side effects are found to occur). The initial clinical dose to be given experimentally to humans will be a tiny fraction of this dose. This preclinical stage is estimated to take from one to two years.

Once animal tests are complete and there is evidence of reasonable safety in animals, drug sponsors can submit an IND plan to the FDA. The IND application outlines plans for human testing in three phases. Included in the IND plan are descriptions of the physical and chemical properties of the drug, its manufacturing process, and results of all preliminary laboratory and animal tests. FDA regulations require animal toxicity testing of at least thirty days duration be completed before human tests are initiated. More animal toxicology testing is required concurrent with human trials to determine possible long-term toxicity during the test animals' lifetimes.[40]

By law, FDA has thirty days to approve the IND or to notify sponsors of a problem. Thereafter, but within an additional thirty day limit, FDA drug evaluators write a comprehensive review to inform the sponsor of deficiencies and to recommend means for correction. After that, according to the report of the Review Panel on New Drug Regulation, the IND process becomes far less structured and defined. The panel cited a lack of any further formal schedule for review unless clinical holds are imposed because of newly emerging safety problems.

Once an IND is approved, the drug sponsor begins the three phases of human clinical testing, as discussed in FDA general guidelines.[41] In phase I, the clinical-pharmacology stage, the drug is given to a small number of healthy volunteer test subjects to determine reasonable drug safety. Drug toxicity and in some cases pharmacology are studied; dynamic and metabolic studies, including those on absorption and excretion, often are carried out during this phase.

FDA guidelines for clinical evaluation suggest the study of from twenty to eighty people in Phase I. These generally should be adults who are either admitted to a hospital or to some other setting that permits close monitoring. As mentioned earlier, initial doses are a fraction of the maximum amount found to produce no serious side effects in animals. If no serious effects are observed, doses are gradually increased. Once these so-called dose-rising studies have established the highest safe dosage desired, prolonged studies at this dose are begun. FDA officials suggest that using a placebo group is useful even in phase I, since as many as 40–50 percent of those on placebo will report side effects. Therefore, a comparison of reported side effects between placebo and drug-administered groups is useful in evaluating possible drug-related toxicity. Occasionally, especially in the case of drugs known to be toxic (for example, anticancer drugs), FDA condones phase I studies in patients only. Concurrent with the phase I clinical trials, long-term animal toxicity studies are undertaken, which usually extend throughout the period of human testing. These studies are designed to determine long-term effects on test animals and on their subsequent generations of offspring. For drugs that affect the reproductive system or are intended for use over long periods of time, these laboratory animal tests are apt to be expensive and lengthy, according to the OTA report on patent term extension.

In phase II, clinical investigation studies, a small number of patients with the disease or condition for which the drug is intended are entered into controlled clinical trials designed to demonstrate effectiveness and relative safety. Patients, usually numbering from 100 to 200, are closely monitored as in phase I. According to the guidelines, they should be free of other serious diseases and should not be receiving other drug therapy if possible. However, patients of the latter type may be included in the late stages of phase II and in phase III studies because they are likely to be representative of the population of patients who will actually take the drug once it is on the market. Phase II studies have been estimated to take about two years.[42]

During phase III, the clinical trial stage, the drug is tested in expanded controlled clinical therapy trials to gather additional evidence of effectiveness for specific indications, and to provide more precise definitions of drug-related adverse effects. No trial size is suggested in the guidelines. These studies have been estimated to take about three years, according to the OTA patent term report.

Finally, according to the FDA guidelines, women of childbearing potential should be excluded from the earliest dose-ranging studies. This refers to any premenopausal female capable of becoming pregnant, including those on contraceptives, but excludes women in institutions such as prisons where pregnancy is considered a highly unlikely event. Women of childbearing potential may be included in the later studies once adequate information on efficacy and relative safety has been obtained, providing certain other segments of FDA animal reproduction test guidelines have been completed.

Testing drugs with a significant potential for use in children should be attempted, according to the guidelines, only when considerable evidence of safety and efficacy in adults has been obtained. This usually occurs late in phase II or early in phase III, although with certain drugs early use in children is considered warranted.

FDA guidelines also cover phase IV, postmarketing clinical trials, to be conducted once the drug is approved by FDA and is available for sale on the market. Circumstances require phase IV testing when:

1. Additional studies are needed to detemrine the incidence of adverse effects or to obtain additional information of some sort.
2. Long-term, large-scale studies are needed to determine the drug's morbidity and mortality effects.
3. Clinical trials have not been adequately studied in a particular patient population, such as children.
4. Further clinical trials are needed to demonstrate efficacy for the proposed indication.

Once the three IND testing phases are complete, the drug sponsor may submit a New Drug Application (NDA) to the FDA for market approval. This huge, expensive document sometimes involves literally truckloads of material, according to some industry officials. By law, the FDA has 180 days to review the application and make a decision. However, the FDA can, and apparently often does, request an extension from the drug sponsor.

The process of seeking FDA approval to include a new indication on the label of a drug already on the market usually is shorter. In this case, FDA requires a supplemental NDA, for which the premarket preclinical and clinical testing requirements are streamlined, pruning the time and costs required. From the standpoint of orphan drugs, however, it is important to note that once drugs are on the market, they can be prescribed by physicians for any use, not just those diseases referred to in the NDA and product label. Therefore, if the new indication is for a rare disease, for instance, drug sponsors may not consider it worthwhile to invest the time and expense necessary to gain FDA approval of the supplemental NDA. When the drug is given for an unapproved indication, optimum doses may not have been worked out and potential adverse effects may not have been fully investigated. Consequently this situation can place patients and physicians at added risk—patients because they may be receiving less-than-fully-tested medicines for their illness, and physicians because their extent of liability is ambiguous. However, the likelihood of serendipity in drug development is increased by research clinicians' experimental use of available drugs for new indications, suggested by hypotheses concerning the drug's possible effect on a specific disease process. This rational approach to testing new uses for drugs has been cited as an important avenue of therapeutic discovery. An accidental, as opposed to rational, observation occasionally takes place when a drug is given to a patient with a particular disease who, coincidentally, also has another condition that unexpectedly responds to the drug therapy. There is even the recent example of an inadvertently bungled home-made narcotic which produced symptoms resembling those of parkinsonism in users, enabling scientists to develop an animal model of the disease, which eventually may lead to improved therapy or prevention of this disorder. In all of these examples, however, added risks are evident. Some industry officials say they are reluctant to include patients with diseases other than the one under study in phase III trials because there is too great a possibility that data will be confounded by these other conditions.

The Law's Effect on Development Time

For new drugs, several industry analysts or members have estimated that the regulatory period (the time from filing the IND to approval of the NDA) averaged about 5 years. Schwartzman, for instance, presents figures showing that for the period 1966–1973, the average period was 4.8 years; the range was between a minimum of 2 and a maximum of 8 years or longer.[43]

Considering just the NDA approval period, FDA took an average of 2.4 years, according to Schwartzman, although the period decreased by 8 months from the late 1960s to the early 1970s. After passage of the 1962 amendments, the preclinical testing period was estimated to have increased from less than 6 months to as much as 12 months. Taken together, these figures suggest that as companies spent more time investigating properties of their drugs, the FDA was able to decrease somewhat the period for review. Nonetheless, the net effect was an increase in development time of almost two-and-one-half years. Schwartzman's figures closely approximated those of other sources, including Harold Clymer's estimate of from 5 to 7 years and Lasagna and Wardell's average of 6.6 years.[44] Lewis Sarett of Merck, when including the preclinical and clinical periods, estimated total R&D time (including regulatory review) at 7 to 10 years.[45] As will be discussed later, although few could argue that establishment of safety and efficacy were not important, the increased development time chipped away important years from the period of patent protection and substantially increased development costs.

The Law's New Costs

Structural changes made at FDA to administer the new law precipitated structural changes within pharmaceutical firms, which were reorganized along lines considered to maximize the firms' ability to get new drugs approved by FDA. Analysts generally contend that the newly structured approval processes instituted in 1962 have resulted in substantially higher costs.[46] The actual extent of the increase is not clear, in part because, as the OTA report emphasizes, absolute R&D costs are difficult to ascertain. Another variable that frustrates analysis is the extent to which other indirect costs are allocated to individual drugs. Still other studies have attempted to provide comprehensive analyses of the financial estimates of drug development costs, profits, and return on investment described next.

By the late 1970s, the pharmaceutical industry was composed of about 1,300 firms, some 750 of which produced prescription drugs. As the OTA report describes, these included generic firms (which produce nonbranded equivalent drugs with aggregate annual sales of about $10 million) and branded drug firms, all of which produce patented drugs, but many of which also produce branded generically equivalent drugs. These companies fall into three general categories. One group consists of large multinational companies, numbering about a dozen domestic firms, which together account for more than one-half of the ethical (prescription) drug sales in the United States, and which conduct an estimated two-thirds of all pharmaceutical research here. The second group consists of medium-sized companies, which are largely domestic, conduct some research, and command about one-quarter of U.S. ethical drug sales. The third group is composed of small companies whose research usually is confined to specific therapeutic areas. Reportedly some of the larger multinational companies are conducting increasingly more of their R&D in other countries because of increased costs of this work here following the 1962 amendments.

One of the lowest estimates of development costs, $2.7 to $4.7 million per new chemical entity (NCE), was reported by the National Science Foundation's Panel on Chemicals and Health in 1973.[47] The figure may be representative for its time, since costs of drugs developed during this early period—when both FDA and industry experienced some confusion about implementation of the law—may not reflect subsequent costs of drugs developed once the regulations and guidelines were well in place.

Schwartzman estimated average discovery (research) cost per NCE at $16.9 million in 1973, and development costs distributed between

NCEs and other products (new combinations and new dosage forms) at $7.5 million. As Schwartzman points out, however, the after-tax costs work out to be about only one-half of this total, or approximately $12.2 million. According to Schwartzman, overall development costs represent an eighteenfold increase over 1960 costs.[48] Hansen projected that a company developing an NCE incurred $54 million in R&D costs in 1976 dollars if R&D expenditures are treated as investment expenditures and are capitalized at 8 percent interest until the date of marketing approval. His calculation included: $30 million in opportunity costs of money alternatively invested at 8 percent interest during the pre-IND period and $24 million in such post-IND costs until the start of drug sales. The total includes aggregate costs of R&D failures; Hodges estimates that seven out of eight drugs that undergo clinical testing never advance to the NDA stage.[49]

The question of anticipated return on these investments then arises. As with costs, return on investment (ROI) is difficult to establish because of the number of underlying assumptions that must be made. As the OTA report on patent term extension describes, major determinants of ROI are R&D costs and expenditures, and subsequent revenues and profit edge. These are interrelated and are also dependent on a host of other factors. Influences on R&D costs, for instance, include inflation, regulatory decisions, and technological changes. Influences on R&D expenditures are cash flow, current revenues, rates of return, and reference projections. Influences on revenues are price and quantity of drug sold, both of which are determined by market size, nature of competition, and patent protection.[50]

As the OTA report illustrates, some profile can be established for factors influencing ROI. Several studies have indicated that firms derive most of their profits from about three leading products. For instance, Virts and Weston's data indicate that 25 percent of drugs on the market account for about 90 percent of sales revenues. Their analysis of 119 NCE's introduced between 1967 and 1976 indicate 25 percent of drugs had average annual wholesales of $21.1 million, whereas the remaining 75 percent of drugs generated an average of only $2.3 million. These figures illustrate the wide range of revenues from sales of different drugs.[51] Companies' reliance on a few market leaders began in the 1950s, as Temin's analysis shows, and this trend has magnified ever since.

Profits in the pharmaceutical industry have been reported to be relatively stable. After-tax rates of return on average stockholders' equity have been consistently high during the period 1956–1979, ranging from a low of 16.7 percent in 1961 to a high of 20.3 percent in the years 1965 and 1966. During this period rates have been consistently higher than those for all manufacturing. As Kefauver's staff had learned, the drug industry's profits were about double those for all manufacturing in the late 1950s and early 1960s, and the industry's profits have remained consistently higher (by about 8 percentage points) throughout the 1970s. Since 1965, revenues from ethical drug sales of U.S.-based firms have grown significantly. The relationship between industry revenues and R&D expenditures has been stable, ranging between 8.2 and 8.8 percent of total sales during the period 1965—1978. Pharmaceutical prices have been rising only slowly since 1967, for a total of 46.1 percent. All industrial prices during this period rose 136.5 percent. But because the quantity of drugs sold has increased, revenues have experienced real growth, all according to the OTA report.

As the OTA report summarizes, several factors favor continued R&D expenditures by industry. These include high, stable profits; improved research techniques, which may decrease costs and improve the rate of product discovery; and the continued pressure for innovation as a means of competition. Nonetheless, according to the report, there is a widespread belief that the return to R&D investment is declining. Schwartzman, for instance, suggests a decrease in return on R&D investment from 1960 to 1967, resulting from sharp development cost increases and a decline in the number of NCEs introduced after passage of the 1962 amendments; but he suggests there has been a rise in expected ROI since 1967, owing in large measure to a growth in market size and lengthening of commercial life of drugs.[52]

The OTA report concludes that there has been a decline in postmarket patent lives from 1966 levels. The average effective patent term was estimated to be less than ten years for drugs approved in 1979 (seventeen years less the years of testing after the patent is granted but before the drug is approved for sale). Since the average for innovations in general is estimated to be between thirteen and seventeen years, the patent term for pharmaceuticals is probably an average of three to seven years less than for other innovations. The OTA report suggests that drug sponsors believe that return on investment is declining. This assumption is based on the decrease in patent terms and on escalating costs of R&D resulting from inflation and stringent testing requirements. These may become even more strict as technology permits finer measures for assessing adverse effects. This belief in falling ROI may prompt drug developers to divert their efforts toward drugs that require relatively shorter R&D

periods, such as drugs for acute rather than chronic administration; to new methods for delivering drug doses; and to patentable modifications of existing drugs according to the OTA report.

Orphan Drugs: One of the Costs

Following passage of the 1962 amendments, increased development costs, decreased patent terms, and the growing belief that return on investment had declined all helped enlarge the group of drugs destined to become orphaned.

Although drugs for rare diseases and unpatentable drugs may have been unattractive to industry prior to the 1962 amendments, these and other orphan-drug categories began to be publicly acknowledged by industry as particularly unwise investments after the amendments were passed.

Official concern about availability of certain drugs was voiced just two years after passage of the amendments, when a committee was formed by the U.S. Public Health Service (PHS) to study the issue. Motivation for forming the committee stemmed from concern that there should be adequate availability of drugs and related products that were not commercially available but were considered by those in the PHS Surgeon-General's Office to be essential to investigational studies or to preserving life in certain unusual emergencies. New needs were seen to be arising in the field of environmental health and in poison control centers. The escalating war in Vietnam also prompted concern that certain drugs would be needed by servicemen there.

As part of the committee's efforts, member companies of the Pharmaceutical Manufacturers Association (PMA) were asked to provide suggestions and a list of drugs currently available as a public service. On the basis of the replies, the Task Force for the Feasibility Study of PHS Facilities for Production of Commercially Non-Available Drugs concluded that PMA member companies were providing ample response to PHS drug needs, and recommended that companies inform the PHS when they discontinue drugs or find new ones of use to the PHS.[53]

In ensuing years, however, concern continued to surface. This was apparent in words and activities at some of the National Institutes of Health (one of the research agencies of the DHHS); at the Centers for Disease Control, which handles development and distribution programs for certain vaccines and anti-infectives; at the

FDA; in medical journal articles; and, at least by 1976, in industry itself.

Most of the industry comments came during a 1976 conference sponsored by the American Enterprise Institute in Washington, D.C., on the Impact of Public Policy on Drug Innovation and Pricing. Henry Grabowski of Duke University drew his concerns from the predictions of Lewis Sarett, then president of Merck, Sharp and Dohme Laboratories, who earlier had performed the company's work in developing cortisone. This was the likely scenario for R&D firms, cautioned Sarett: (1) a relative shift from research to development (three major companies had shown a 15–25 percent budget shift from research to development in the past ten years); (2) a shift away from me-too drug research; and (3) increased emphasis on epidemiologically important diseases. Rare diseases, according to Grabowski's account, would be accorded nominal surveillance and, within some economic limits, would be combatted by service drugs produced as a social responsibility of industry firms. Moreover, the emphasis on drug safety would encourage companies to concentrate R&D dollars on acute-term drugs, rather than on chronically administered drugs whose safety is more difficult and time-consuming to establish.[54] For instance, Jacob Stucki of Upjohn has estimated that chronic disease drugs require about twice as long to develop as those for short-term use.[55] Grabowsky's message was this: Companies will be concentrating not on research but on development of drugs for short-term use in large markets.

Barry Bloom, a vice-president for research at Pfizer, shared Sarett's view of the plight of drugs for chronic use. He asserted that the industry had not been making progress at a rate commensurate with current knowledge and resources on major crippling and lethal diseases afflicting modern-day society. As evidence of declining interest in chronic-disease drugs, Bloom presented data showing a gradual decrease in NCEs for use in chronic diseases, dropping from twenty-two NCEs introduced in the 1955–1959 period to eight NCEs introduced in the 1970–1974 period. Although there had been a corresponding drop in all NCE introductions between these two periods as a result of the 1962 amendments, Bloom of Pfizer suggested that drugs for treating chronic degenerative diseases of the cardiovascular and pulmonary systems, as well as those for treating inflammatory and metabolic diseases, were particularly lacking.[56]

Similarly, the comments of Merck's Lewis Sarett concerning emphasis on drugs intended for large markets, as opposed to those for rare diseases, were reiterated by James Russo of SmithKline Beckman (a former PMA president) who wrote that firms do devote most research money to diseases afflicting large numbers of patients, asserting that inflation in research costs and increasing federal regulation sometimes renders it less than worthwhile to manufacture and market a drug the cost of which could run as high as $100 a pill.[57]

Although Sarett's scenario did not refer directly to the unprofitable economics of unpatentable drugs, Roy Vagelos, the current president of Merck, Sharp and Dohme Laboratories, did so. Vagelos told the House Judiciary Subcommittee on Courts, Civil Liberties and the Administration of Justice that a major factor in his decisions to commit R&D funds is the extent to which the work can and will have patent protection, according to the OTA report. More recently, Jacob Stucki of Upjohn reiterated that point, saying that patent status is considered at the outset of any development decisions. Work on a drug may proceed while patent status is determined, but drugs without patent protection are not likely candidates for NDAs.[58]

At the American Enterprise Institute meeting, Armistead Lee had commented that patent protection for drugs for rare diseases was relatively unimportant because other firms were unlikely to market a competing drug for the same rare disease. Using the example of Lederle's rabies vaccine, Lee suggested Lederle had a monopoly without monopoly power (patent) for this reason.[59] Although the extent to which such a natural monopoly may exist for unpatentable drugs useful in treating rare diseases has been neither demonstrated nor questioned, data on drug sales in the 1960s and on NCEs developed from the mid-1960s to the mid-1970s indicate unpatentable drugs constituted a fraction of total drugs available. William Comanor, then of Harvard, reported in 1964 that more than two-thirds of all prescription drug sales were for patented drugs.[60] Schwartzman mentioned data showing that only 15 percent of the ninety-five NCEs introduced between 1966 and 1973 were not protected by product patents.[61] Clearly, unpatentable drugs, whether for small or large markets, constitute their own orphan category.

Patent protection took on added significance in 1975, when the government established the MAC (maximum allowable cost) program for drug reimbursement under Medicare. Under MAC, reimbursement for multiple-source drugs was to be limited to the lowest cost at which chemically equivalent drugs are generally available, plus a reasonable dispensing fee. Medicare patients whose physicians prescribe a brand-name or generic drug that exceeds the MAC price must make up the difference themselves. Exceptions are granted if physicians certify in writing that the higher-priced drug is medically necessary. MAC was anticipated to save Medicare 5 to 8 percent a year. According to generic manufacturers, however, only about twenty-two drugs are included on the MAC list to date. Thus the provision has not benefited the generic producers or Medicare to any great extent.

As William Comanor, now at the Federal Trade Commission, noted in his discussion of the nature of competition and financing in the pharmaceutical industry, the past dozen or so years have seen numerous economic studies on these topics. The studies point in different directions, presumably because they are based on differing assumptions. He therefore cited the need to develop a common framework within which to consider how the results fit together.[62] Although generalizations about price competition, costs, and ROI are sometimes contradictory and open to challenge, it does appear that, relative to other drugs, orphan drugs are at a distinct disadvantage when development discussions turn to finances.

Industry executives were not alone in expressing concern over problems of potentially unprofitable but medically important drugs. J. Richard Crout, then director of the FDA Bureau of Drugs, emphasized at the 1976 American Enterprise Institute meeting that the problem was growing and was expected to increase as more drugs came off patent.[63] The FDA, prompted by the concern of academic and federal research scientists, already had initiated one task force to look into the problem (to be discussed in later chapters). Journal articles and editorials detailing difficulties in development and approval for certain categories of orphan drugs, especially drugs for rare diseases, were raising some of the major scientific, ethical, and legal aspects of the problem.

This was still an insider's dialogue, whose major points were little known outside the medical research community. But patients and their families, though generally unaware of the nature of market and regulatory constraints, knew there had been no drugs developed that might help them, and some began to try to find out why.

Commenting on the problem in general, Rawlins wrote in a 1977 *British Medical Journal* article that research into drugs for rare diseases was at a standstill—partly, he suggested, because academic pharmacologists had concentrated on elucidating fundamental principles of drug action while scorning the idea they should undertake drug discovery.[64] At about the same time, a *Lancet* editorial dramatized the gap between drug development by academic scientists and their subsequent inability to find market sponsors.[65] In an article in the *New England Journal of Medicine*, research clinician Melvin Van Woert detailed his futile efforts to find a commercial sponsor interested in further developing L-5HTP for use in the rare neurological disorder termed *intention myoclonus.*[66] This stimulated a response from James Russo (described earlier) and from Thomas Althius of Pfizer, who acknowledged that, although there were problems requiring a cooperative spirit among industry, universities, and the FDA, industry had not been ignoring the plight of unprofitable drugs but, rather, had been providing more than forty such drugs as a public service.[67]

Despite the absence of systematic new planning or legislation, the NIH now had several drug development programs firmly in place. The FDA, primarily under the leadership of Marion Finkel (then deputy director of the Bureau of Drugs), prompted DHHS to create a second interagency task force to explore the problems and make recommendations to that department.

By the late 1970s, readers of *Science* and the *Wall Street Journal* alike were coming to realize that the new techniques of molecular-genetics and recombinant-DNA research and monoclonal antibody probes were synonymous with new approaches to drug therapy, which could become big winners, both medically and financially. These technologies resided primarily at the academic institutions where they were developed. At once it seemed as though all the earlier industrial transformations—technological, legal, and organizational—were on the threshold of further radical change. No one knew whether orphan drugs again would be among the casualties. As the next two chapters describe, several federal drug programs were firmly in place, although they differed in philosophy, practice, and funding levels and had grown up in the absence of coordinated planning and legislation. They had evolved out of a recognition that orphan drugs were financial thorns in the flesh of the pharmaceutical industry.

Notes

1. Louis Lasagna, "Who Will Adopt the Orphan Drugs?" *Regulation* 3(6)(1979):27–32.

2. Lewis Thomas, *The Youngest Science* (New York: Viking Press, 1983), pp. 13–15.

3. James H. Young, *The Toadstool Millionaires* (Princeton, N.J.: Princeton University Press, 1961).

4. Milton Silverman and Philip R. Lee, *Pills, Profits & Politics* (Berkeley: University of California Press, 1974), p. 2.

5. Ibid., p. 3.

6. *Patent-Term Extension and the Pharmaceutical Industry* (Washington D.C.: Office of Technology Assessment, 1981), pp. 50–51.

7. Silverman and Lee, *Pills,* pp. 26–27.

8. Upton Sinclair, *The Jungle,* (New York: Doubleday, Page and Company, 1906).

9. Peter Temin, "Technology, Regulation and Market Structure in the Modern Pharmaceutical Industry," *Bell Journal of Economics, 10*(2)(Autumn 1979): 427–446.

10. Thomas, *Youngest Science,* p. 21.

11. Ibid., pp. 32–35.

12. Silverman and Lee, *Pills,* p. 4.

13. Thomas, *Youngest Science,* p. 35.

14. Silverman and Lee, *Pills,* pp. 86–87.

15. B. Abrams, "Commentary on Therapeutics and Government 1776–1976," *Clinical Pharmacology and Therapeutics 20*(1)(July 1976): 1–5.

16. Silverman and Lee, *Pills,* p. 87.

17. Temin, "Technology," pp. 434–435.

18. Richard Harris, *The Real Voice* (New York: Macmillan, 1964), pp. 21–25.

19. Temin, "Technology," pp. 435–441.

20. Silverman and Lee, *Pills,* p. 6.

21. Temin, "Technology," pp. 441–442.

22. Harris, *Real Voice,* pp. 26–30.

23. Temin, "Technology," pp. 443–445.

24.. Ibid., p. 442; David Schwartzman, *Innovation in the Pharmaceutical Industry* (Baltimore, Md.: Johns Hopkins University Press, 1976), pp. 106–107.

25. *OTA Patent-Term Report,* pp. 18–19, 30.

26. Harris, *Real Voice,* pp. 64, 90.

27. Donald Kennedy, "A Calm Look at Drug Lag," *Journal of the American Medical Association (JAMA) 239*(5)(January 30, 1978): 423–426.

28. *OTA Patent-Term Report,* p. 26.

29. Barry Bloom, "Socially Optimal Results from Drug Research," in S. Martin and E. Link, eds., *Impact of Public Policy on Drug Pricing and Innovation* (Washington, D.C.: American University, 1976), pp. 344–370.

30. Harris, *Real Voice,* pp. 27–30.

31. Ibid., p. 17.

32. Ibid., pp. 56–62.

33. Ibid., p. 95.

34. D.D. Anderson, "Who Owns the Regulators?" *Wharton Magazine* 4(4)(Summer 1980).

35. Harris, *Real Voice,* pp. 181–193.

36. Silverman and Lee, *Pills,* pp. 88–97.

37. Harris, *Real Voice,* p. 200.

38. Ibid, pp. 205–206.

39. *Review Panel on New Drug Regulation* (Washington, D.C., Department of Health, Education and Welfare, 1977).

40. Schwartzman, *Innovation,* pp. 14, 33–47, 57–59.

41. *General Considerations for the Clinical Evaluation of Drugs* (Washington, D.C.: U.S. Government Printing Office, 1977), pp. 1–11.

42. *OTA Patent-Term Report*, p. 14.

43. Schwartzman, *Innovation*, pp. 174–176.

44. Harold Clymer, "The Changing Costs of Pharmaceutical Innovation," in J. Cooper, ed., *The Economics of Drug Innovation* (Washington, D.C.: American University, 1970); Louis Lasagna and William Wardell, *An Analysis of Drug Development Involving New Chemical Entities Sponsored by U.S. Owned Companies, 1962–1974* (Washington D.C.: American Enterprise Institute, 1974).

45. Lewis Sarett, "FDA Regulations and Their Influence on Future R&D," *Research Management* 3(1974):19–20.

46. Schwartzman, *Innovation*, pp. 136–299; R.W. Hansen, "The Pharmaceutical Development Process: Estimates of Development Costs and Times and Effects of Proposed Regulatory Changes," in Robert Chien, ed., *Issues in Pharmaceutical Economics* (Lexington, Mass.: Lexington Books, 1980), pp. 151–181; *OTA Patent-Term Report*, pp. 25–36.

47. *Report of the Panel on Chemicals and Health of the President's Science Advisory Committee* (Washington, D.C.: U.S. Government Printing Office, 1973), NSF 73-500.

48. Schwartzman, *Innovation*, p. 149.

49. Hansen, "Pharmaceutical Development," pp. 160–181; R.M. Hodges, "Research and Regulations," *Analytical Chemistry*, 50(6)(May 1978):534a.

50. *OTA Patent-Term Report*, pp. 13, 33.

51. J.R. Virts and J.F. Weston, *"Expectations and Allocation of R&D Resources,"* in R.B. Helms, ed., *Drugs and Health* (Washington, D.C.: American Enterprise Institute for Public Policy Research, 1980), pp. 21–45.

52. Schwartzman, *Innovation*, pp. 143–152.

53. Carolyn Asbury, "A Systems Approach to Orphan Drugs" (Ann Arbor, Mich.: University Microfilms International, 1982).

54. Henry Grabowski, J. Vernon, and L. Thomas, "The Effects of Regulatory Policy on the Incentives to Innovate: An International Comparative Analysis," in S. Mitchell and E. Link, eds., *The Impact of Public Policy in Drug Innovation and Pricing* (Washington D.C.: American University, 1976), pp. 47–82.

55. Jacob Stucki, Upjohn, presentation at Mount Sinai Medical Center meeting, March 1984.

56. Barry Bloom, "Socially Optimal Results," pp. 344–370.

57. James Russo, "Profitable and Non-profitable Drugs," *New England Journal of Medicine* 299(1978):156.

58. Stucki, presentation.

59. A.M. Lee, "Comparative Approaches to Cost Constraints in Pharmaceutical Benefits Programs," in S. Mitchell and E. Link, eds., *The Impact of Public Policy on Drug Innovation and Pricing* (Washington, D.C.: American Unviersity, 1976).

60. William S. Comanor, "Research and Competitive Product Differ-

entiation inthe Pharmaceutical Industry in the United States," *Economica* (November 1964).

61. Schwartzman, *Innovation*, p. 167.

62. William Comanor, "Competition in the Pharmaceutical Industry," in Robert Chien, ed., *Issues in Pharmaceutical Economics* (Lexington, Mass.: Lexington Books, 1980), pp. 67–68.

63. J. Richard Crout, "New Drug Regulation and its Impact on Innovation," in Mitchell and Link, eds., *Impact*, pp. 241–317.

64. M. Rawlins, "No Utopia Yet," *British Medical Journal* 2(1076)(October 1977).

65. "Drugs for Rare Diseases," (editorial), *Lancet* 2(7970)(1976):835–836.

66. Melvin Van Woert, "Profitable and Non-profitable Drugs," *New England Journal of Medicine* 298(16)(1978):903–906.

67. Thomas Althius, "Orphan Drugs: Debunking a Myth," *New England Journal of Medicine* 303(17)(October 23, 1980):1004–1005.

3
Orphan Drugs as Wards of the State: The Federal Role

The medical and pharmaceutical historian James Harvey Young characterized the government's role in medical drugs as threefold: *generator* (discoverer and developer), *guarantor* (protector of patents), and *guardian* (consumer protector through safety and efficacy regulations).[1] Federal orphan-drug activities of the past three decades have been essentially expansions of those roles. During this time, the government accelerated drug R&D activities, became liability insurer in one instance, and sought to provide regulatory flexibility in orphan-drug approval. Rather than being part of some overall plan, however, these events occurred more by what Redman terms "legislative dance" than by design.[2]

Generator

The generator function gained momentum in the midst of the drug boom of the mid-1950s. Despite the spate of new drug introductions, cancer treatment then remained virtually the same as in the 1930s. Progress had come to a standstill despite some apparently promising leads in academic settings in the 1940s. The National Cancer Institute (NCI) asked Congress for authorization to pursue these leads, and Congress responded with new dollars for anticancer drug research. This entry of NIH into drug R&D was not new. In fact, scientists at the Hygienic Laboratory of the Marine Hospital Service, which eventually became the National Institutes of Health (NIH), developed vaccines for Rocky Mountain spotted fever and typhus in the early 1900s. During World War II, in cooperation with the pharmaceutical industry, this laboratory developed chloroquine for treating malaria, and participated in efforts led by Vannevar Bush to develop mass-production methods for penicillin.

The new aspect of the NCI program was a coalescence of federal and voluntary health agencies appealing to Congress for increased public dollars for drug-related R&D. This practice was reenacted many times during the next two decades by different NIH institutes and voluntary organizations, on behalf of increased spending for development of such diverse measures as contraceptives, vaccines and other biologicals, and drugs for the treatment of epilepsy. These general programs were augmented by individual grantee-initiated drug projects (those proposed by university scientists seeking federal research grants). When John Adams, a vice-president of the Pharmaceutical Manufacturer's Association (PMA), estimated that industry had spent approximately $40 million on forty orphan-drug products by 1969, Edward Burger of the Office of the President's Science Advisor was estimating that the federal government had spent approximately $657 million on drug-related R&D between 1960 and 1975.[3] To some extent, both government and industry's orphan-drug dollars were being spent on testing for possible new uses of drugs already developed and marketed; this was particularly true of federal efforts. But the NCI and, later, other NIH institutes were mounting major programs for development of new drugs for rare diseases.

Guarantor

The guarantor function of government grew as a result of these R&D efforts. The NCI program introduced new legal and ethical questions concerning proprietary rights to products or production methods developed with federal funds. NCI officials found that trade-secret status of data and patent guarantees threatened the fragile negotiations for joint-venture agreements with pharmaceutical firms. Their solution was to make exemptions to industry by administrative action, thereby paving the way for the NCI program as well as others that followed.

Meanwhile, court decisions in liability cases were translating medical catastrophes into financial ones. Vaccines and drugs for women of childbearing age were consigned to orphan status. In 1976 these liability judgments culminated in a new role for government as guarantor: assumption of responsibility for liability claims in the swine flu immunization program.

Guardian

Finally, the guardian function of government was somewhat streamlined in response to repeated requests from academic and NIH scientists involved in orphan-drug development. These individuals felt they were at a disadvantage in trying to grapple with a regulatory process designed for drug sponsorship by large organizations. Despite isolated instances of administrative flexibility in certain FDA drug review and approval situations, by the mid-1970s the FDA had developed no systematic means for dealing with the varied problems posed by premarket requirements of orphan drugs.

In aggregate, it seemed that orphan drugs had become wards of a state unprepared to accept them.

The NCI Program

The outlook for patients with cancer has improved significantly since 1955, the beginning of the NCI drug development program, according to Vincent DeVita and his colleagues at the NCI. At the start of the program, the overall cure rate for all cancers was 33 percent, attributable primarily to surgery, to the use of X-rays to treat tumors that could not be seen or felt, to blood transfusions and antibiotics, and finally to a few new drugs. By 1977, 60 percent of the 700,000 patients diagnosed with various forms of cancer (exclusive of skin and in situ cervical cancers) were candidates for systemic treatment. For instance, according to the NCI scientists, 71 percent of new cases are found to have localized tumors. Of these, 40 percent can expect to remain tumor-free with the use of surgery or radiotherapy alone; the remaining 31 percent can be expected to develop recurrent tumors if only local treatment is used. Now NCI scientists believe that more than one-half of these patients should receive postoperative treatment systemically with drugs recently developed for use in these common cancers (including breast, ovarian, bladder, colon, and head and neck cancers).

Moreover, of the remaining 200,000 patients with metastatic as opposed to localized tumors, nearly one-half can expect to benefit from existing chemotherapy. Finally, according to the NCI scientists, widespread application of cancer therapies has led to a marked decrease in mortality from cancer nationally since 1954 in those aged forty-five and under. The NCI can take substantial credit for this record. It has participated in developing and/or clinically evaluating every antineoplastic drug available today in the United States.[4]

Answers to the question of why and how NCI became involved provide one of the most systematic and comprehensive illustrations of the evolving federal role in orphan-drug development and availability. The *why*, as answered by DeVita and colleagues, is attributed to industry's failure to exploit the early successes observed with antitumor drugs because of the high costs and low rate of return involved in underwriting antitumor drug research.

The three early successes mentioned by DeVita and colleagues include nitrogen mustard, antifol aminopterin, and methotrexate. Nitrogen mustard, introduced in 1943, seemed effective in treating Hodgkins disease and other lymphomas. That excitement was short-lived because all patients relapsed. Shortly thereafter, Sidney Farber realized the antitumor effect of antifol aminopterin in treating acute childhood leukemia; by 1950, methotrexate, a similar drug, was introduced for use in choriocarcinoma of the uterus. Both drugs eventually were found to be capable of inducing complete remission in many patients.

The answer to *how* the NCI program began and flourished is more complicated. It illustrates the potential for combining technological innovation with effective planning and politics. Briefly, the Cancer Chemotherapy Program began as a small, grant-oriented effort to develop antileukemia agents. The program was based on the three drugs just mentioned and on the use of transplantable tumors in syngeneic rodents as a system for testing new drugs. This formed the technological basis of the NCI drug development program.

The NCI's advisory council had strongly urged the institute to take over the antitumor agent screening program initially developed at Sloan-Kettering Memorial Institute in New York. The number of compounds submitted for testing had exceeded Sloan-Kettering's capacity for screening. The council's advice was in keeping with suggestions made after passage of the 1937 National Cancer Act that the NCI conduct or support animal research aimed at discovery of new therapeutic agents. Encouraged by dramatic early results in treating leukemia and choriocarcinoma, in 1955 the U.S. Congress authorized $5 million to establish a Cancer Drug Development Program at the NCI. Congress had witnessed spectacular results from industry's targeted program to develop antibiotics; cancer might yield to the same kind of concentrated effort. According to DeVita and colleagues, much of the research conducted between 1955 and 1970 was devoted to testing one hypothesis—namely, that drugs could, by themselves, cure patients with metastatic cancer. According to the authors, by 1970 that hypothesis had been proved. The current research emphasis, according to these authors, is on testing new approaches to multimodal therapy—using all known effective treatments at the time of initial diagnosis—in patients who can be expected to develop recurrent tumors after surgery or radiation treatment for apparently localized tumor. These include the 200,000 patients with breast, ovarian, bladder, colon, and head and neck cancers.

Within three years, the NCI Cancer Drug Development Program had grown into a massive, $35 million industrial program funded through contracts, with grants used only for coordinated clinical trials, according to two major figures in the NCI, Gordon Zubrod and Saul Schepartz and colleagues.[5] The elaboration that follows provides a glimpse into the intricate issues raised by the potential cooperation between public and private sectors.

Establishing Proprietary Arrangements

NCI developed eight goals. Among them were identifying neglected research areas, developing protocols for chemotherapeutic agents, and developing a basis for voluntary cooperative studies. This last goal turned out to be a formidable task.

The NCI convened a meeting with industry representatives to request that promising chemicals be sent for screening. Despite a perception by NCI officials of industry interest, if not enthusiasm, only one company—Upjohn—submitted compounds. During this first year almost all of the 5,000 compounds submitted came from academic or government scientists.

Thereafter, according to Zubrod and his colleagues, marketplace strategies were introduced into NCI's approach. NCI redrafted its agreement to provide for trade-secret status of data. The agreement also provided that NCI would not seek assignment of patent rights from suppliers. Under the new provisions, when NCI employees were coinventors with a supplier, the government and the supplier would share rights to the invention. Each situation was to be resolved by negotiations between the surgeon-general and the supplier. After a disappointing start, market safeguards now stood to clear the way for a long-term joint industry-government endeavor. Industry soon was submitting more than half the compounds screened. The 1958 drug development budget was $35 million, solidly built on precedents for preserving the trade-secret status of data and on patent protection.

Effects of the Program

Seven different means for joint development of drugs were invoked in ensuing years, according to DeVita's comprehensive article on the NCI program. They were:

1. Total development and marketing by the pharmaceutical company following discovery of activity by NCI screening (pipobroman).
2. Total drug development and sponsorship of clinical trials by NCI, with industry involvement only at the marketing step (nitrosoureas and DTIC).
3. Cooperative development with major scientific and financial contribution by NCI (cytosine arabinoside and mithramycin).
4. Drugs developed by a U.S. pharmaceutical company, with NCI clinical testing (vinblastine, vincristine).
5. Foreign pharmaceutical company development of drugs with NCI sponsorship of U.S. clinical trials (adriamycin and bleomycin).
6. NCI development, production, and clinical evaluation of special forms of commercially available drugs (high-dose methotrexate, parenteral forms of melphalan, 6-mercaptopurine, and thioguanine).
7. Discovery of the optimal dose by NCI both for drugs developed after the program's start and for those marketed prior to NCI involvement.

Moreover, there are five different levels of contractual interactions between NCI and industry, ranging from contracts to perform selected tasks, to contracts awarded solely for marketing an NCI-developed drug, to contracts to carry out an entire series of development steps.

A total of twenty anticancer drugs have been fully developed since the NCI program began in 1955. Twelve were sponsored directly by NCI; the remaining eight were evaluated by NCI in collaboration with industry-sponsored clinical trials.[6]

The next National Cancer Act was passed in 1971, with the hope that curing cancer, like sending a man to the moon, depended primarily on allocating enough money. Congress's optimism had been fueled by the impressive record compiled by NCI; since inception of the Institute's program, the number of anticancer drugs on the market had nearly doubled. Despite contrary advice by NCI officials that technology might not be as ready for the cancer mission as it had been for the space mission, the budget for clinical trials of experimental cancer therapies (including drugs) rose dramatically to $117.5 million by 1980.

Costs

NCI officials estimate that the cost of preclinical development of an antitumor drug (including acquisition, screening, formulation, and toxicology) ranges from slightly more than $200,000 to nearly $400,000 depending (in ascending order of expense) on whether the agent is synthesized, fermented, or derived from plants. Screening synthetic compounds and natural products that prove to be inactive in preliminary tests costs about $125 per compound; testing an active compound through the complete panel of tumors costs about $5,300.[7] Total costs for developing a single drug, including clinical trials, range from $1 million to several million dollars.[8]

NCI's screening approach has changed with time, and officials are not yet certain of the ramifications of the changes. During the 1960s the "fractional kill hypothesis" was revived by Drs. Skipper, Schabel, and colleagues at Southern Research Institute. It formed the biological basis for the treatment protocols, enabling researchers to quantify the relationship between drug dose, tumor response, and tumor volume. Until the mid-1970s screening was done in an empirical random process in rodents bearing the L1210 leukemia as well as various other tumors. By 1971, about the time of the passage of the National Cancer Act, officials were satisfied that the model discriminated between active drugs and inactive ones, but suspected it was failing to uncover some important new classes of drugs, since the screening system was designed using only drugs that were clinically available in the 1950s. In 1975 NCI turned to a screening method that tested drugs against matched pairs of tumors of the same organ system. Concomitantly, the number of chemicals screened decreased from 40,000 to 15,000 annually. Although final evaluation of the new screening approach is still in the future, DeVita and colleagues note that the number of new active drugs coming out of the program compares favorably with that under the old system. Screening fewer compounds also means spending less money at this preliminary stage of the process.

Unpatentable Orphans

Within this range of development activity, DeVita reserves the designation of *orphan* drugs for those that cannot be protected by patent. The combination of small and nonexclusive markets has made industry unwilling to invest time and manpower in such drugs as o,p'DDD, dimethyl triazenoimidazole carboxamide (DTIC), as well as the nitrosoureas BCNU and CCNU. In the case of o,p'DDD, an informal agreement was reached whereby a given company agreed to market the drug after NCI agreed to carry out any further studies FDA might require. For the remaining three drugs, NCI negotiated no-cost contracts with pharmaceutical companies, selected through competitive bidding. These companies assembled the necessary data to take the drug through the NDA process.[9]

Requirements Uncoordinated with FDA

Problems with late entry by companies into this process could be substantial, as described in 1981 by William Hubbard, Jr., president of the Upjohn Company, in testimony before Congress. Hubbard said that Upjohn discovered streptozotocin (Zanosar) and first evaluated it as a potential antibiotic. After an anticancer screen suggested it had some biologic activity, Upjohn made the compound available to the NCI, which conducted animal pharmacology, toxicology, drug formulation, and clinical trials. After the NCI published evidence of streptozotocin efficacy in pancreatic islet cell carcinoma in 1973, Upjohn decided the drug—the only agent known to have potential therapeutic benefit for the 300 people each year who develop this unusual cancer—should be approved and marketed. However, said Hubbard, Upjohn had wrongly assumed that clinical and toxicological results obtained by NCI would be acceptable for NDA approval by the FDA. Instead, Upjohn's investigators had to collect original case reports from physicians participating in the NCI study, and reanalyze all data published as a result of the NCI contract efforts. The NDA, which had been submitted in 1976, had not yet been approved at the time of Hubbard's testimony in 1981. Upjohn was then engaged in discussions with FDA about manufacturing techniques and control procedures. It was difficult for Upjohn officials to understand that all of this duplication of effort was necessary to protect the public from inappropriate availability of unsafe or ineffective drugs.[10]

Hubbard concluded that data required by NCI were fully adequate for making prudent scientific judgments on drug safety and efficacy but that there was a lack of fit between these requirements and the legal ones dictated by FDA regulations. According to NCI officials, this problem has occurred frequently with companies other than Upjohn as well. Recently, NCI renewed attempts to have companies become involved prospectively. If companies themselves filed the IND, perhaps there would be greater opportunity to coordinate NCI requirements with those of the FDA. Officials at other NIH institutes similarly have found discrepancies in NIH and FDA data requirements to be a major problem. This relates primarily to a failure of interagency coordination, a situation that could be readily improved.

A Record of Achievements

Despite such difficulties, no one disputes the remarkable achievements of the NCI program. For instance, market introduction of anticancer drugs has remained relatively stable for the past two decades while that for other classes of drugs has declined, according to a report by the Center for the Study of Drug Development at the University of Rochester. An average of about one to two NDAs for anticancer NCEs are approved each year. The NCI files an average of seven INDs per year. In contrast, anticancer agents accounted for only 2 percent of industry NCEs studied in humans from 1963 to 1976, according to the Rochester study report. The study concludes that the relatively high rate of NCI introduction of INDs has balanced out industry's relatively low rate compared to its activities in antibacterial, endocrine, and cardiovascular IND investigations. Industry's involvement with anticancer drugs was seen as similar to that for other orphan categories such as antifertility drugs, motor-system drugs (anti-parkinson agents and muscle relaxants), and central depressant agents (hypnotic sedatives and antiepileptic agents).[11] Finally, the study indicates that the proportion of INDs terminated for reasons related to anticipated small market was not as high for anticancer agents (25 percent) as for antibacterial agents (39 percent). The lower fail rate of anticancer INDs occurs in part because much of the work on many of the anticancer agents is done by NCI prior to investment by a pharmaceutical firm, whereas most of the work on antibacterial agents requires total funding by pharmaceutical firms.

In aggregate, there is compelling evidence that the NCI drug development program has played a strong role in advances in cancer chemotherapy during the past three decades. The precedents set by NCI with regard to trade-secret status of data and patent rights facilitated new efforts by other NIH institutes to build formal drug development programs, most notably those involving contraceptives, immunobiologics (including vaccines and antiparasitic agents), anticonvulsants for epilepsy, and drugs used to combat substance abuse.

Varied NIH Policies

Before describing these other formal programs, it is useful to note that each institute developed its own approach and philosophy independently, guided by no formal NIH-wide policy and tempered only by budgetary constraints.

For example, the NCI budget was orders of magnitude larger than those of other institutes after passage of the 1971 National Cancer Act. The NCI drug development program was a major beneficiary of the act. Through what is designated a Group C class of drugs, the NCI has made its drugs available to physicians for their patients as a free service. The designation was created for these anticancer drugs in recognition that safety and efficacy had been reasonably demonstrated; although the drug was not officially on the market, it was no longer purely experimental, either.

The National Institute of Neurological and Communicative Disorders and Stroke (NINCDS), with a substantially smaller budget, decided it was not authorized to provide money to grantees to purchase drug supplies apart from those specifically related to the research and covered by the research grant. Therefore, for instance, Melvin Van Woert was unable to obtain funds from the institute to buy supplies of L-5HTP to treat his patients with action myoclonus after the grant funds for studying the action of the drug had run out.

The divisive issue of whether to fund only research or to include "patient service" as part of the mission has confronted many of the NIH institutes. It was a major dilemma for the National Heart, Lung and Blood Institute (NHLBI) during deliberations concerning funding of the artificial heart program; and it had been a major philosophical, scientific, and medical issue for the National Institute of Arthritis, Diabetic, Digestive, and Kidney Diseases (NIADDK) as officials debated its appropriate role in the development of kidney dialysis programs.

On a smaller scale than the heart and kidney deliberations, the National Institute of Allergy and Infectious Diseases (NIAID) decided without much hesitation to provide, free of charge, a supply of sera matched for histocompatability antigen type on special trays for use in kidney and bone marrow transplants, at an annual cost of $300,000. Institute officials decided to supply the service for three reasons: (1) insufficient market for industry interest; (2) short supply of materials; and (3) inflexible FDA requirements of uniform standards for different sera, which, according to Institute officials, further eroded industrial interest.[12] The establishment of formal NIH programs, in addition to the NCI drug development effort forced officials to make explicit decisions concerning service versus research funding, and to define the nature of the collaboration they desired to have with industry on drug programs.

The Epilepsy Drug Program

Impetus for the formally established Antiepileptic Drug Development (ADD) program came from both scientific and political sources. The program, devised by the Epilepsy Branch at NINCDS (the Neurology Institute), initially was intended to develop clinical trial methodologies and then to conduct clinical trials of antiepileptic agents already available in other countries. Later, as the NCI had done, the Epilepsy Branch developed a screening system for identifying agents with potential anticonvulsant activity.

The ADD program was created in 1966 in response to a report to the Surgeon-General's Public Health Service Advisory Committee on the Epilepsies. The report said many firms had no new antiepileptic drugs under development for marketing since previous antiepileptic INDs had been deemed by FDA reviewers to have inadequately established efficacy and had been denied approval. Industry officials cited prohibitive development costs with expected low marketing return to be the single most important disincentive. Since 1960, according to Ronald Krall and his colleagues at NINCDS, only three new antiepileptic drugs had been marketed. In contrast with the ease with which anticonvulsants can be identified, commented the authors, development into marketable drugs is complicated by corporate assessment of their commercial value. Contributing to the assessment was the difficulty of demonstrating efficacy, and the high incidence of side effects occurring with chronic administration. The authors also cited industry's presumption of small market potential (a view the NINCDS scientists did not share) and the "environment" governing relations between industry and the FDA.[13]

Antiepileptic drug development clearly was curtailed following passage of the 1962 Kefauver-Harris amendments. Most of the information on that situation comes from a report issued by the ADD program.[14] Prior to 1960, sixteen drugs were marketed for epilepsy. The first (potassium bromide) was discovered more than a hundred years before phenobarbital was introduced in 1912. A quarter century later, phenytoin became the first nonsedative antiepileptic available. The additional thirteen drugs were introduced during the next twenty years. After the 1962 amendments, however, only one new drug was introduced in the next decade, despite the large number of patients whose seizures were not optimally controlled by existing drugs. Thus the NINCDS program was begun.

A pressing need was to develop clinical trial methodologies. The type of seizure is the major determinant of the appropriate drug, but often seizure type is difficult to discern from patient history. Using video recording and telemetered electroencephalography, adapted from National Aeronautics and Space Administration (NASA) instrumentation to monitor astronauts during space flight, NINCDS scientists soon were able to identify and categorize seizure types by monitoring patients for prolonged periods.

Thereafter, the ADD program initiated clinical trials of four drugs marketed in other countries, culminating in FDA approval of carbamazepine (Tegretol) in 1974, clonazepam (Clonopin) in 1975, valproic acid (Depakene) in 1978, and clorazepate in 1981 for adjunctive treatment in epilepsy. All four drugs had commercial sponsors throughout the NDA process and were subsequently marketed.

Difficult clinical and ethical questions faced ADD scientists. For instance, what is an appropriate control population? Since it is unethical to remove a patient's previously prescribed antiepileptic drug to test whether seizure severity or frequency increases or decreases with the test drug, do appropriate control populations exist? Or can only patients with poorly controlled seizures be studied? Some seizure types are uncommon, making it hard to assemble a test population. Moreover, since the disorder varies substantially among patients, diagnostic and evaluation criteria cannot be applied generally. These problems make for lengthy and extremely detailed clinical trials. Finally, since 75 percent of all patients with epilepsy have their first seizure before the age of eighteen, often test participants must be teenagers or children.

Determining that the United States should not depend solely on agents initially developed abroad, ADD scientists looked into the factors constraining epilepsy drug development here. They found that academic medicinal chemists did not have access to pharmacologic testing of anticonvulsants in a timely fashion. ADD scientists then followed NCI's example. The ADD program began a screening program in 1975. This was facilitated—in addition to clinical trial methodologies—by development of a model of partial seizures in monkeys. Although the relevance of animal models to human epilepsy is indirect, they are valuable in distinguishing fundamental seizure types.

Two years after ADD set up the screening system, the congressionally mandated Commission for the Control of Epilepsy and Its Consequences recommended continued federal funding for new drug development and advised the ADD program to expand this animal-testing screen for potential new drugs with promise. A toxicology and pharmacology capability in rats and dogs was established in 1980.

Program scientists adopted a policy of urging pharmaceutical firms to make a financial commitment to any of their compounds entering this stage of development. ADD program officials also helped university researchers find pharmaceutical industry sponsors who might participate in funding at this point.

Toxicology and pharmacology testing, which takes about one to two years, is estimated by ADD officials to cost $250,000 to $700,000 per drug. It includes, in addition to toxicology, the other tests routinely required by FDA (carcinogenicity, effects on reproduction and embryonic development, effects of formulation on absorption and metabolism, and possible specific organ toxicity).

To date, according to program director Roger Porter, two new compounds have passed this phase and are being contracted out for clinical testing. These are the first home-grown epilepsy drug candidates since 1960, and both have pharmaeutical firm sponsors.

Academic scientists have provided more than one-half (60 percent) of compounds screened. ADD scientists speculate that identification of promising, biologically active compounds might accelerate submissions to ten times the current rate. Finally, just as the NCI grew concerned that screening methods based on drug technology of earlier years might not be sufficient in view of current advances, ADD scientists, like those at NCI, have adopted a new screening model based on recent neurochemical theory. Still, as the program summary states, coordinating government-sponsored research with federal regulatory requirements or with the needs of commercial sponsors of new drugs continues to be "challenging."

Contraceptive-Agent Development

Echoing its concern over the lack of cancer drugs, Congress also enacted legislation on contraceptive agents, though on a much smaller scale. Through an amendment to the Public Health Act proposed by then Senator Joseph Tydings (D-Md.), contraceptive-agent development was designated as a priority area, with funds earmarked to establish a Center for Population Research in the National Institute of Child Health and Human Development (NICHD). The center, which spends more than $7 million annually for basic studies in this area, has been involved in five investigational contraceptive-agent projects.

Apparently, safety concerns over long-term use of contraceptives by women of childbearing age have seriously dampened industry interest in this area. Both long-term testing requirements and uncertain litigation possibilities loom as disincentives, according to industry officials.

The recent battle over Upjohn's attempts to market Depo-Provera in the United States demonstrates the reality of these uncertainties. Depo-Provera, injected intramuscularly, provides three months of contraceptive protection. It has been used for as long as twenty years and is used currently by about 10 million women in countries other than the United States (where it has not been approved as a contraceptive). Reportedly, FDA has not approved the NDA because the drug, shown to be carcinogenic in animals, is intended for long-term use in healthy individuals. According to FDA official Robert Temple, Upjohn has not discredited the animal studies, has not demonstrated the absence of carcinogenic risk through persuasive human studies; and has not shown that some people need the drug desperately despite the possible risks.[15] FDA approval for use in the United States is important to Upjohn not only for the potential domestic market but also because many other countries allow the sale only of FDA-approved drugs.

Finally, with regard to male contraceptive agents, apparently the need for government funding for development has arisen because industry anticipates a relative lack of interest on the part of the intended male market.

Cardiovascular-Drug Development

Although the National Heart, Lung and Blood Institute (NHLBI) has no formal congressionally mandated drug development program, it budgeted $21 million in 1978 for major clinical trials. These included: an aspirin–myocardial infarction study; a trial of propranolol, an agent for angina and for cardiac arrhythmias; a multicenter trial on limitation of heart attack severity using propranolol and hyaluronidase; and a study on prevention of neonatal respiratory distress syndrome using antenatal administration of corticosteroids.[16] Although most of these drugs are intended for relatively large numbers of people, most also are not patented, a factor that dims an otherwise optimistic projected financial return. Essentially, these studies represent clinical trials for new uses of drugs already marketed. Perhaps because the drug studies were not organized as a unified program, as were the cancer and epilepsy drug activities, Heart Institute officials reported difficulty in determining the number and type of drug studies that are being conducted with institute support. Even so, the institute's contribution has been significant.

For instance, propranolol was one of 5 cholesterol-lowering drugs which were being prescribed for heart attack patients even though there had been no significant proof they improved chances for survival. NHLBI studied the drugs, and found that propranolol was the only effective one. In fact the NHLBI study on propranolol so convincingly established its efficacy in improving the chances for survival in heart attack patients that clinical trials were halted for ethical reasons and the experimental therapy became standard practice. Propranolol has been credited with lowering heart attack mortality by 26 percent.[17]

Drugs for Treating Substance Abuse

Developing drugs to treat drug addiction or abuse has become a major effort of the National Institute on Drug Abuse (NIDA). The program is an outgrowth of the 1960s, a time when government realized, as one NIDA official commented, a need to treat "junkies."

Pharmaceutical companies apparently have shied away from this area of drug development for several reasons. First, if substance abuse drugs themselves are addictive, they must be carefully tracked. This requires substantial paperwork. For instance, methadone, used to treat heroin addiction, requires careful monitoring of its distribution and use. Second, intended users of the drug therapy may reject the idea; this shrinks the market size. Third, informed consent for conducting clinical trials may pose substantial liability questions, and safety problems may be especially difficult, particularly if the drug therapy is itself addicting. This also may mean restricting drug use to males through excluding use by women of childbearing age, further shrinking the potential market (the postmenopausal female market is estimated to be small). Fourth, companies may be reluctant to risk unfavorable public relations by producing drugs for drug abusers. Finally, exacerbating the situation is the prospect that the drug may not be patentable.

All these conditions, in fact, exist for LAAM (L-alpha-acetyl-methadol), a long-acting methadone drug and a major orphan product of NIDA. The institute recently submitted the NDA on LAAM to FDA, representing one of the few times a federal institute or agency, instead of a pharmaceutical firm, has applied for marketing approval. NIDA's filing was not done by choice. Rather, it is the culmination of a long and frustrating experience for NIDA, which is not over yet.

LAAM is a narcotic, as addicting as methadone. NIDA officials expected that LAAM, since it is long-acting, would confer a major advantage over methadone since users would need to come to LAAM clinics only two or three times weekly instead of daily as is required with methadone. The dropout rate with methadone has been attributed in part to the need for a daily visit to the clinic, and take-home methadone has obvious control problems. LAAM has been available for more than thirty years, so the drug no longer has patent protection. According to one NIDA official, the drug was "the only game in town," and it has been a $2 million line item in NIDA's budget for about ten years.

The initial contract for LAAM was awarded to a new firm headed by John Whysner, an M.D., Ph.D. who previously had worked at NIH and then at the Special Action Office on Drug Abuse, established by the White House. Whysner's firm had competed successfully against one other bidder for the NIDA contract to test LAAM. Well into clinical trials, however, a newspaper column by Jack Anderson raised questions concerning the appropriateness of the contract, suggesting that Whysner's former position at the Drug Abuse Office and as consultant to NIDA on the LAAM project conferred unfair advantage in the competition.[18] The Anderson column suggested this was one of many inappropriate contract dealings of NIDA. Whysner and NIDA officials countered that his firm's bid won on merits, but in the ensuing "Whysnergate" controversy, he relinquished rights to the contract through a settlement with NIDA and, following in Gauguin's footsteps, reportedly left for Tahiti to learn wood-carving for a few months before returning to Washington.

The Anderson column also described alleged abuses by two Los Angeles LAAM clinics in their practices for gaining informed consent from clinical-trial participants, who were previous heroin users attempting to convert to the LAAM substitute. The column reported that several participants had sworn they were subjected to coercion and harassment to sign up for the program. NIDA filed the NDA about two and a half years ago. Because there was no commercial manufacturer of LAAM (supplies were being obtained through bulk manufacture by a university pharmacy department), however, FDA could not approve the application without the Good Manufacturing Practices component. NIDA then engaged a firm to compile data, but, according to a NIDA official, FDA did not accept it because of prior problems in dealing with the firm. NIDA then generated replacement data, but FDA still was not satisfied with the data format. Finally, FDA determined that the drug could not be considered orphaned because it had a sponsor, albeit a federal one. Apparently

NIDA still has several hundred users on LAAM, which can continue to be dispensed because it falls under a permanent IND (a so-called Compassionate IND).

NIDA officials had proceeded with the drug on the assumption that securing a company's interest in marketing LAAM, once approved, would require a demonstration of market potential. Since the LAAM IND covers use only in males, NIDA officials estimated a potential U.S. market of 10,000, based on the assumption that about 10 percent of males on methadone would cross over to LAAM. However, difficulty in finding a commercial sponsor was compounded by the fact that LAAM was not protected by a product patent. Under the Freedom of Information Act, clinical data on LAAM would be generally available to firms. Therefore, NIDA could not issue a restrictive license to a specific firm to market the drug. More than six years after Whysner's firm took the first steps toward marketing LAAM, the drug's future remains uncertain.

The Drug Abuse Institute also has been involved in development of three other drugs, one of them related to LAAM. Naltrexone, needed for reversing a LAAM overdose, was subjected to carcinogenic studies by NIDA. A company with an interest in developing narcotic drugs to treat pain has begun studies on naltrexone for pain control and as a LAAM antagonist. NIDA also has an IND on Bufenorphine, a synthetic narcotic marketed in Britain (at 0.4 mg) for treating pain. At a somewhat higher dose its effect changes to that of a narcotic antagonist. The drug is patented and presents no overdosing problems—two factors that increase its commercial attractiveness. NIDA anticipates that marketing this drug, as opposed to LAAM, should entail fewer headaches for the agency.

The third drug under investigation by NIDA is clonidine, marketed as Catapres for its anti-hypertensive action. It may have potential in detoxifying methadone and heroin users. Since the drug is marketed already as an antihypertensive, NIDA's task involves gaining FDA approval for including this new use in the drug's labeling. Otherwise, according to NIDA officials, the liability problems could be quite complex if the drug is prescribed for a use not specifically approved by FDA.

Liability issues are of concern to NIDA, especially those concerning its own drug, LAAM. For instance, NIDA officials question whether—if the institute pays for R&D and applies for the NDA—NIDA can be held liable for possible adverse effects. Could clinical-trial participants bring suits against NIDA, and even perhaps against individual researchers? If so, and if a conflict arose between defending individual researchers and NIDA, which group would DHHS lawyers represent? Could users, once the drug is on the market under licenses to pharmaceutical firms, win suits against NIDA, against the firms, or both? Is NIDA liable for suits concerning package insert or labeling? According to one NIDA official, many of the issues are not even defined, much less settled, in any way.

These liability uncertainties are not unique to NIDA. All federal research agencies have the same or similar questions with respect to drug projects, although few have had to apply for an NDA directly, as NIDA has done with LAAM. Another therapeutic area prone to liability difficulties is vaccines. Two federal agencies have been heavily involved in vaccine development and distribution; the Centers for Disease Control (CDC) and the National Institute of Allergy and Infectious Diseases (NIAID).

Immunobiologicals, Vaccines, and Antiparasitics

The federal government, in cooperation with a number of pharmaceutical firms, has played a major role in the development, refinement, and distribution of vaccines. These activities have been carried out primarily by the Centers for Disease Control (CDC) and the National Institute of Allergy and Infectious Diseases (NIAID).

Vaccines constitute an orphan-drug category in themselves, as is readily acknowledged by the FDA's Bureau of Biologics which is responsible for their approval.[19] Liability is a major contributing factor, but a host of other constraints also have relegated vaccines to orphan status. As described by Roy Widdus, who is directing a comprehensive assessment by the National Academy of Sciences (NAS) on barriers to vaccine development, the problems are legion:

1. The target disease may be rare in this country (limited sales).
2. Vaccine manufacturers face difficulties in identifying target populations (those at high risk for the disease) and therefore in being able to provide vaccine in a timely manner.
3. Large-scale human clinical tests are required. This is expensive.
4. Vaccines have high production costs and require separate production facilities.
5. Quality control is extremely difficult and expensive.
6. Routine vaccine (especially viral vaccine) is difficult to produce.
7. Manufacturers face uncertainty about what the CDC Immuni-

zation Practices Advisory Committee will recommend concerning the vaccine's use, based on committee members' assessment of the vaccine's safety and efficacy. According to Widdas, these recommendations have disappointed manufacturers on some occasions.[20]

According to an Office of Technology Assessment (OTA) study, these factors—especially low profits coupled with extensive federal regulations and widely publicized court cases—have caused the number of vaccine manufacturers to drop precipitously from thirty-seven to eighteen in the past twelve years. Moreover, in 1979 only eight companies were actively producing vaccines.[21] Despite all these disincentives, Merck has maintained a major program in vaccines and has a strong public-service reputation for doing so. Similarly, other companies that have kept vaccines in their product line as a public service include American Home Products (Wyeth), Lederle, Pfizer, Merrell-Dow, Parke-Davis, and Cutter Laboratories. Nevertheless, as the OTA report concludes, the problems are formidable.

As Schwartzman indicates, at the turn of the century effective vaccines had been developed for typhoid fever, cholera, and plague, as well as for anthrax and rabies.[22] Silverman and Lee credit government agencies with research leading to the development and/or evaluation of improved vaccines for prevention of mumps, measles, German measles, and various respiratory infections.[23] Recent additions to that list include vaccines in which NIAID has been involved, including those for hepatitis B, pneumococcal pneumonia, and meningococcal A and B infections.

NIAID's role can be considered a natural evolution of the early federal development of vaccine for Rocky Mountain spotted fever and typhus waged by the predecessor to NIH, the Hygienic Laboratory. A recent assessment by NIAID indicated the institute had been involved with fourteen vaccines or immunobiologicals that now have NDAs, including the three mentioned earlier. NIAID also is studying twenty-six immunobiologicals in IND status.

Concurrently, CDC has been distributing twelve immunobiologicals. The agency was the source or producer of two of these and held the IND for five that were produced primarily by drug firms (Parke-Davis and Merrell-National, now Merrell-Dow). CDC also distributes fourteen parasitic-disease drugs manufactured by a number of international firms for use in the United States, as part of a parasitic-disease drug program begun in 1967.

In addition to CDC's role in developing vaccines and antiparasitics, it maintains a large distribution effort for rarely needed biologicals that are not readily available in this country, as well as programs for childhood and influenza immunizations. Both these programs will be discussed.

Distribution of Rarely Needed Biologicals

CDC is concerned with two types of products: those that are approved for marketing in the United States but are rarely needed and therefore are difficult to obtain; and those that are not commercially available in this country but are provided to CDC by drug sponsors under special provisions used by FDA.

As with the Group C designation of anticancer drugs, these rarely used biologicals and drugs are maintained in Compassionate IND or Treatment IND status. Usually drugs available under these mechanisms are those that are widely used in other areas of the world and are required by international travelers returning to this country (those in military service, and tourists) or by international visitors here. Since teratogenic, mutagenic, and long-term effects of drugs have not been fully evaluated, none is recommended for use in pregnant women or in children under two years of age, according to Sandra Ford of CDC.[24]

CDC provides these products to physicians on request; the physicians fill out appropriate forms required by CDC and FDA, and have their patients sign consent forms required by FDA. CDC uses the program as one means of maintaining epidemiologic surveillance of specific diseases in this country. In general, the cooperative arrangement between CDC and drug firms has been considered an effective means of ensuring drug availability while monitoring and containing the potential for epidemics.

The program's effectiveness is threatened occasionally by steadily rising requests for CDC's biologicals. Increased travel, greater awareness of CDC's program on the part of physicians and pharmacists, and improved diagnosis and reporting of parasitic infections all have contributed to this surge in demand.

In some instances, an overwhelming number of demands have strained CDC supplies. One of the most striking illustrations is the case of pentamidine isethionate, manufactured by the British firm May & Baker Company. Although the drug's primary international use has been in treating African trypanosomiasis (sleeping sickness), it also has been found to be effective in cases of pneumocystis carinii, a type of pneumonia sometimes encountered in immunosuppressed patients following organ transplantations and cancer chemotherapy.

As the number of requests for the drug to treat patients in these two therapeutic situations approached 12,000 per year, CDC advised that the drug should be licensed in this country, even if it meant stretching the regulations a bit. At the time, fairly extensive phase I and phase II studies had been conducted by foreign researchers, and CDC had published some phase III studies.[25]

CDC continued to rely on British supplies, but it encountered a profound problem in meeting the demand created by the current epidemic of AIDS (acquired immune deficiency syndrome). Cases of AIDS reportedly have doubled every three months, and pneumocystis carinii is one of the major diseases afflicting these immunodeficient patients. Recently, the Generic Manufacturers Industry Association (GPIA) and member company Zenith stepped in to ensure adequate supplies of the drug from May & Baker Company for use by CDC until U.S. production of the drug is approved by FDA.[26] CDC has appealed to the pharmaceutical industry to complete necessary tests for FDA approval so that the agency does not have to continue to incur a six-month waiting period for delivery of May & Baker Company shipments.

Childhood and Influenza Vaccination Programs

Vaccines are of two general types: those for childhood immunizations (polio, diphtheria, measles, rubella, tetanus, whooping cough, and mumps) and those for influenza immunizations, used by people of all ages but often especially recommended for those over sixty-five years of age and those with certain medical conditions who can be seriously affected by influenza. Childhood vaccines remain essentially the same from year to year, but influenza vaccines differ annually depending on the biological properties of the virus. Therefore, the efficacy of vaccines for use against influenza virus, which is likened to a moving target, can be more difficult to establish.[27]

As Walter Dowdle of CDC stressed in congressional testimony, firms not only have difficulties distributing 20 million doses of vaccine per year, but also end up having to buy back about 10 percent of the unused vaccine at the end of the year. Then, when there are shortages in other years, the firms are blamed.[28]

CDC provides grants for state and local childhood immunization programs. The agency purchases vaccine, assists health departments in setting up programs, and conducts epidemiologic surveillance. Every state has a mandatory vaccine immunization law for children entering school. As a result, childhood immunization rates are estimated at 90 percent for all routine vaccines.[29] About one-half of these children are vaccinated through these CDC grant-funded programs, the other half through private physicians.[30] The major difficulty in the present program lies in vaccinating the remaining 10 percent of children, and also in reaching children earlier—before they enter the school system—especially in large, low-income urban areas and in rural areas.

Vaccine costs rose 30 percent in 1982.[31] In 1981, CDC spent $24 million on grants to state programs.[32] According to Office of Technology Assessment officials, the childhood immunization programs were found to be not only cost-effective but actually cost-saving; they provide net health benefits and reduce net medical costs.[33]

OTA studies indicated that influenza vaccine programs also were cost-effective.[34] CDC's Dowdle cautioned that annual variations in influenza epidemic intensity and populations affected make cost-effectiveness analyses difficult. Wide confidence limits are required to calculate direct medical expenses and estimates of efficacy. Nonetheless, according to Dowdle, three studies on cost-effectiveness of immunization on those sixty-five years of age and over support OTA's general conclusions.[35]

CDC provided direct support for the 1977 swine flu immunization program, one that had precedent-setting liability consequences for the federal government (discussed in the next section). Since the 1977 program, the CDC has not provided financial support for influenza immunization programs, but does (1) provide technical advice on vaccine formulation and potency, (2) license manufacturers, (3) maintain quality control, (4) monitor for significant vaccine-related adverse reactions, (5) evaluate safety and efficacy of vaccines, and (6) conduct and support research leading to improved vaccines and more effective influenza control.[36]

Liability issues are significant for vaccines as well as for other types of drugs, including those intended for long-term use or for use by pregnant women, children, or drug abusers—"orphan" groups at which many of the federal drug development programs have been aimed. These liability concerns are not unfounded, as the next section describes.

Before addressing the liability issue, it is worth noting here that the CDC vaccine and antiparasitic agent programs allude to another orphan category—namely, drugs for developing nations. Policymakers and pharmaceutical firms have tended to consider issues related to drugs for developing nations separately from those affecting domestic orphan-drug development. Indeed, many of the problems are very different. These issues were discussed recently by health-care providers from developing nations attending a conference on drugs for primary health care sponsored by the Harvard University School of Public Health. They emphasized problems with drug distribution stemming from lack of adequate transportation infrastructures and lack of health-care providers to staff clinics, especially in rural areas. Often national health budgets are not considered sufficient to pay for large amounts of pharmaceuticals. Political and trade policies may change abruptly. Additionally, drugs represent only one element in improving public health; they need to be accompanied by other preventive health measures such as sanitation and adequate supplies of nutritional food. Rural areas seldom are served by doctors, and too few health-care providers are trained to administer drugs. Many nations do not adhere to patent laws, a practice that discourages pharmaceutical industry drug R&D on diseases endemic to developing nations. These are just a few of the complex and interrelated issues. The recent book by Silverman and Lee, *Prescriptions for Death: The Drugging of the Third World*, details these and many other drug problems in developing nations, including shipping them outdated drugs, providing little information on adverse effects, and embellishing the expected therapeutic effects.[37]

As Myron Schultz, an official of the CDC's antiparasitic disease service emphasizes, parasitic diseases are the "cancers" of developing nations. Yet total international research expenditures on tropical infectious disease annually reached only $30 million U.S. dollars in 1975, whereas one "developed" country alone spends nine times that much on cancer research.[38] A similar theme emerged during a World Health Organization (WHO) International Medical Sciences Roundtable, where it was reported that the possibility of developing suitable vaccines against parasitic diseases has not been explored even though a degree of natural immunity is in many cases a well-established sequel to infection.[39] Although CDC maintains a program on antiparasitic-agent development and distribution, these international orphan drug needs have remained outside the direct policies of CDC.

The Swine Flu Program and Liability

In the midst of federal efforts in 1976 to prevent a possible swine flu pandemic similar to the one that claimed 500,000 U.S. lives in 1918, the federal government indemnified swine flu vaccine manufacturers from product liability. Through P.L. 94-380, the government set a precedent as liability insurer.

The legislation was prompted by an announcement from the four vaccine suppliers (Parke-Davis; Merrell National; Wyeth; and Merck, Sharpe and Dohme) that casualty insurers had refused to provide coverage for the mass immunization program. Since the vaccine was intended to reach 200 million people in the United States, insurers said they were unable to rate the risk of vaccine administration to virtually the entire population.

According to Neustadt and Fineberg of Yale, who pieced together the chronology of events leading up to passage of the law, casualty insurers were concerned primarily with anticipated overhead costs: Since insurers were obliged to defend their clients (vaccine manufacturers) in court, they feared too many of the 200 million doses would result in poorly adjusted claims, which in turn would lead to lawsuits and high overhead costs.

The American Insurance Association identified three constraints to insuring the vaccine manufacturers. First, the legal climate was too unsettled to permit actuarial calculation. Second, the casualty insurance industry had lost more than $7 billion worldwide underwriting product liability in 1974 and 1975. Third, insurers felt the federal government should defend all claims.[40]

Vaccines containing inactivated influenza virus have been marketed here since the 1940s, and high-risk populations (including those over 65 years of age; those with chronic heart, pulmonary, renal, or metabolic diseases or anemia; and those who have immune deficiencies) have been advised to receive immunization. Usually only about 20 percent of people in these high-risk groups request or receive vaccine.[41] According to CDC's Dowdle, prior to the 1976 swine flu immunization program, influenza vaccines had not been shown to be associated with any significant adverse reactions other than local soreness and redness; nevertheless, there was the possibility that a small number of individuals might experience rare side effects as a consequence of infection.[42]

The insurers' concerns were not groundless. They were based on early judicial rulings that pharmaceutical firms could be held liable for adverse effects without proof of negligence as a necessary prerequisite. The insurers' decision was reinforced by a more recent judicial ruling that manufacturers could be held liable for failing to warn adequately of risks. This latter ruling, according to Neustadt and Fineberg, was the major deterrent to commercial coverage of the swine flu vaccine.

Legal Precedents

Henry Grabowski and colleagues at Duke University, pointing to Cutter Laboratory's experience, emphasized the growing importance of liability in pharmaceutical firms' decisions.[43] Cutter allegedly manufactured a batch of virulent, instead of killed, Salk polio vaccine. Thereafter, the firm was held liable for the ensuing cases of polio, according to Nathanson and Langmuir's carefully documented account of the so-called Cutter incident.

By Nathanson and Langmuir's description, certain lots of Cutter Laboratories' Salk (killed-virus) polio vaccine contained residual virulent virus. Thereafter, according to the researchers, sixty people who were vaccinated and eighty-nine family contacts developed poliomyelitis clearly related to the vaccine. The case prompted a reconsideration of the extent of implied warranty. Cutter Laboratories were held legally responsible for the cases, and fifty-four of the sixty suits were settled for a total of more than $3 million. As the researchers explain, this sum grossly exceeded Cutter's insurance coverage of $2 million.[44]

This precedent-setting decision, holding the manufacturer liable without fault in tort and warranty, was a red flag for vaccine manufacturers. Even in instances where vaccines are not faulty, a small percentage of children receiving childhood vaccines do develop reactions—some strong, a few fatal. Usually, according to Frederick C. Robbins, president of the National Academy of Sciences Institute of Medicine, this is due to a hereditary defect in immune capability. The instances are rare, according to Robbins—about one in many millions of doses. Approximately 6 children developed polio associated with the vaccine in 1981; and while the smallpox vaccine was still in use—before the disease was eradicated through worldwide vaccination—about 100 children per year would experience vaccine-related reactions.[45] It is estimated that about 1 in 310,000 infants or young children per year develop serious reactions to the diphtheria, pertussis, typhoid (DPT) vaccine.[46]

A second major precedent set in another vaccine case sealed this category's fate as a liability problem. About nine years after the Cutter Laboratories decision, the case of *Reyes* v. *Wyeth* (498 F2nd 1264) in 1974 held the manufacturer liable for failing to extend an adequate warning of risk of harm. In this case, the circuit court upheld a jury award of $200,000 to the parents of an eight-month-old infant who had contracted polio after receiving the Wyeth-manufactured Sabin live-virus attenuated (weakened) polio vaccine. As Neustadt and Fineberg put it, this was the outcome even though the company had included a printed form with adequate warning in vaccine shipment cartons, and even though experts had testified that the case was not vaccine-related. The Supreme Court refused to hear the case and the award thus held. The precedent that Wyeth had the duty to advise all those vaccinated of potential harm from the vaccine was seen by the PMA, according to Joseph Stetler, PMA president at the time, as posing an absolutely impossible task—one that manufacturers and their commercial insurers were not willing to take on with the swine flu program, with its intended goal of vaccinating 200 million people.[47]

Swine Flu Vaccine Liability Arrangements

A CDC official raised the concern that liability problems might drive vaccine manufacturers out of business. He spoke out just days before the first cases of respiratory disease at Fort Dix, New Jersey, were reported and later identified from throat swabs as swine-type influenza A viruses. Following a DHEW decision to mount a nationwide immunization program to prevent the possibility of another swine flu pandemic, the government entered into what was to become a tortuous exercise of trying to develop a means for legal protection of commercial vaccine manufacturers. Those attempts vacillated from administrative to legislative initiatives. Based on the Cutter and Reyes precedents, commercial insurers had refused to insure the four potential vaccine manufacturers. As Neustadt and Fineberg note, the insurers were in business to spread risk, not take it.

Jolted into action by the sudden outbreak in Philadelphia of what later was termed Legionnaires' disease but initially was reported as possibly the first swine flu fatalities, Congress moved to enact liabiliity legislation. A legislative formula using the Tort Claims Act as a model was worked out by DHEW general counsel William Howard Taft IV and Congressman Paul Rogers (then chairman of the House Subcommittee on Health and the Environment).

The legislation specified that any claim arising from the swine flu program should be filed against the government, but the government had the right to sue for compensation from other participants. If negligence occurred on the part of manufacturers, they could be sued by the government, but they would be insured for this eventuality by commercial insurers. There was no need to indemnify. Manufacturers were freed from the duty to warn. Manufacturers and insurers incurred no overhead costs. Instead, civil servants would process claims and defend against groundless suits. Neither manufacturers nor insurers would have to worry about suits arising from failure to warn of harm, or about suits claiming an adverse effect had occurred even though negligence had not been a contributing factor. In these cases, the government would assume liability responsibility.[48] Thereafter, the government developed a consent form, which attempted to provide adequate warning about possible adverse effects from swine flu immunization.

Slightly more than two months and 40,000,000 inoculations after the official start of the swine flu immunization program, it came to an abrupt halt. Reports transmitted to the CDC from health departments in ten states noted fifty-four cases of Guillain-Barré syndrome (GBS); of these, according to Neustadt and Fineberg, thirty vaccinees had received swine flu shots anywhere from one to thirty days before onset of symptoms.

GBS is a self-limited but often severe paralytic polyneuritis that is most commonly triggered by viral infections. There are about 2,500 new cases in the United States each year. Approximately 30 percent of GBS patients will require a respirator during the course of the illness, which usually runs several weeks. Recovery generally is good, although about 10 percent of patients are left with residual effects. Mortality is low, about 3–4 percent of patients.[49]

Influenza infection and vaccinations generally are not important trigger agents for GBS, according to an epidemiological study by Lawrence Schonberger and colleagues at CDC. Ordinarily, the crude annual incidence rate for GBS ranges from 0.6 to 1.9 per 100,000 population. The A/New Jersey influenza vaccine administered in the 1976–1977 program, however, represented a major exception, according to the CDC epidemiologists, with the occurrence of just under 1 excess case of GBS per 100,000 vaccinees.[50]

Since negligence in manufacturing the vaccine was not found to be a factor, the Justice Department was the sole responsible legal entity. To date, the Justice Department has received claims totaling $3 billion. After vaccine-associated cases of GBS began to be reported to CDC, that agency and the National Institute of Allergy and Infectious Diseases (NIAID), which together had been instrumental in proposing the massive immunization plan, advised curtailing the effort pending examination of the GBS factor. CDC requested that diagnostic criteria be established to aid its current and future epidemiologic surveillance of GBS. A four-member ad hoc committee of neurologists expert in GBS, appointed by the two national neurology professional associations and convenened by the National Institute of Neurological and Communicative Disorders and Stroke (NINCDS), characterized the disorder for this purpose. The committee, chaired by Arthur K. Asbury of the University of Pennsylvania, drew up guidelines stating that the basis for diagnosis was descriptive, resting on recognition of clinical patterns and on laboratory and electrodiagnostic criteria. The problem, according to the committee report, was not in recognizing a typical case, but in knowing the boundaries by which the core disorder is delimited.[51] According to Asbury, the guidelines, though developed as an epidemiologic tool, frequently have been used as a basis for ruling on the suits brought before the courts.[52]

Neustadt and Fineberg characterized the swine flu program as the first one on the "slippery" end of the disease spectrum. In contrast to well-established federal immunization targets such as measles, polio or smallpox, where causes, symptoms, and vaccination risks are well understood, flu is a slippery disease. Immunization is short-lived, since antigenic shifts in the virus can occur annually. In the instance of the swine flu program, vaccination risks were not well understood. Finally, delineating vaccine-associated GBS from that which occurs naturally, and defining the diagnostic limits of the disorder, all caused some difficulty in a small number of the vaccine-associated GBS claims.

Amid speculation on how the swine flu experience will affect the future of federal flu immunization programs, the government's course during the first post–swine flu vaccination years suggests that subsequent efforts against flu will be aimed primarily at high-risk groups. Yet the federal presence in vaccine research, development, distribution, and now liability insurance indicates that vaccines are another orphan category in need of further attention.

For instance, legislation introduced in the 98th Congress by Senator Paula Hawkins (R-Fla.) sought to increase federal responsibility for adverse effects from the childhood vaccine program. The legislation proposed that the government compile a list of known vaccine-associated adverse effects. When those effects occur in vaccinated children, the government could be required to provide compensation. The DHHS assistant secretary for health, Edward Brandt, Jr., has commented that although the problem is an important one the bill as currently written is unworkable.[53]

Liability for Drugs for Women of Childbearing Age

Vaccines are not uniquely subject to major liability problems. Shortly after the Cutter incident, according to Grabowski, contraceptive agents joined vaccines as liability targets. A.H. Robins, manufacturer of the popular Dalkon Shield intrauterine contraceptive, was named in thousands of claims asserting device-related infections, uterine perforations, spontaneous abortions, and other problems.[54] By 1976, Robins had made payments of $3 million; by Grabowski's count, more than 3,000 claims were still pending. A recent update reports that the company and its insurer in aggregate have paid out approximately $179 million in about 6,500 claims, averaging $22,500 per claim. The company directly incurred expenses and settlements related to the shield of $18.7 million in 1983, $7.1 million in 1982, and $3.3 million in 1981.[55] Edwin Chen of the *Los Angeles Times* writes that there were 165 claims remaining against Robins in San Francisco alone in 1982, asking for a total of more than $6 billion (including punitive damages).[56]

A few recent examples of liability claims may illustrate the complexities encountered with this category of orphan drug. One is the case of Upjohn's Depo-Provera, which, as discussed earlier, has not received FDA approval for use as a contraceptive in this country because of agency officials' concern over its safety. The drug is now the subject of a class action suit by the National Women's Health Network on behalf of women whom the network says have suffered from the drug's unauthorized use, according to a *Los Angeles Times* report. Depo-Provera is approved for use in this country in kidney and endometrial cancers, but it does not have FDA approval for use as a contraceptive because animal studies have linked it to cervical and breast cancers in test animals. Because the drug is approved for sale and is on the market, however, individual doctors can prescribe it as a contraceptive. Upjohn's vice-president for pharmaceutical research has said that his company persists in seeking FDA approval for the proposed contraceptive use because there is a demonstrable need, which Upjohn feels a responsibility to meet. Additionally, the company is convinced that, among the hormonal contraceptives, the drug has outstanding efficacy and safety. The National Women's Health Network has maintained a register of Depo-Provera users since 1979, containing reports of 529 women who say they experienced adverse side effects. One effect cited by some women was breast tumor, a side effect demonstrated in animals that persuaded the FDA to deny approval of the drug. Other adverse effects cited included menstrual irregularities, mental depression, weight gain, infertility, blood clots, high blood pressure, and swelling of limbs.[57] Many of these side effects have been reported by users of other contraceptives that are approved. Additionally, this information does not derive from controlled clinical trials, making the true incidence of drug-related effects difficult to assess. The case illustrates problems for producers and consumers alike with drugs whose safety may be difficult to establish. It also illustrates the uncertain position in which physicians are placed when prescribing drugs for uses not authorized to be included in the drug's labeling.

DES, or diethyl-stilbesterol, illustrates the risks pregnant women may be taking in using any drugs during pregnancy, and the liability difficulties that can be encountered by companies manufacturing drugs for use specifically in this so-called orphan population. DES, a synthetic hormone, was used by as many as 2 million pregnant women from 1941 to 1971 to prevent miscarriages. Doctors observed that daughters of women who took DES during pregnancy were at a higher risk of developing vaginal cancer than the comparable control population (daughters of women who did not take the drug during pregnancy); initial studies also suggested there might be a higher incidence of sterility in males born to women taking the drug. In this instance, teratogenic effects in children born to these women were not evident until the children were in their teens. Such long-term effects are of course difficult—if not impossible—to detect in premarket studies of limited duration.

The situation was complicated further by the fact that several companies manufactured DES. A 1980 California Supreme Court decision ruled that all companies could be held liable for damages, to be apportioned on the basis of market share. The U.S. Supreme Court refused to review the decision. Adding to the complexity of determining liability responsibility is the fact that each state has its own liability laws. A coalition of business and insurance companies now is asking for increased federal regulation in product liability litigation, but this issue is far from resolved. Chen reports the coalition's chief complaint is the extent of differences among states in the statutes of limitation and in liability standards.

Also at issue are the two schools of thought concerning the onset of liability responsibility. One school holds that liability starts once exposure has occurred, even though the exposure or its effect is not discovered until after an insurance policy has expired. The other holds that liability begins only when a disease has manifested itself, so that insurers whose policies have ended by the time a relationship is demonstrated are no longer responsible. The issue is receiving increased attention from environmental (particularly asbestos) and occupational (such as black lung disease) hazard cases. The issues are complicated and, according to Chen, the stakes are growing. For instance, South Carolina law professor David Owen found that as of 1976 the largest product liability punitive award approved by an appellate court in a case involving fradulent marketing of a dangerous drug was $250,000, whereas today multimillion-dollar awards are almost common.[58]

As described earlier, FDA guidelines discourage testing of drugs in women of childbearing age and in children until the drug is almost fully developed and initial indications of safety are well documented. Therefore, many useful drugs are not specifically approved for use in children or in women of childbearing age because of potential unforeseen adverse effects. Here again, however, once the drugs are on the market, individual doctors can prescribe them for their patients in these two categories—even though information on contraindications for these users is lacking. In the past, FDA also discouraged testing of drugs in persons over sixty-five years of age, because older persons may have conditions requiring the use of other medical drugs, thereby raising the likelihood of drug interactions. Robert Temple of FDA has said that the agency may have discouraged drug testing in older patients in the 1970s, when guidelines for clinical testing were first drawn up by FDA as an aid to pharmaceutical firms, but the agency no longer holds that view. In fact, FDA officials consider it important for clinical trials to include older patients because they are becoming an increasingly larger segment of medical drug users.[59]

Pneumococcal vaccine summarizes many of the problems discussed in this section. It demonstrates the unique complexities occurring with a product that combines factors related to vaccines with those relating to drugs intended to be used by older people and by people in developing nations. In this instance, a debate over proof of efficacy, not safety, is the issue.

The vaccine, developed by Robert Austrian of the University of Pennsylvania and marketed by Merck in 1977, has met with only modest enthusiasm by physicians. Prior to the advent of antibiotics, pneumococcal infections were one of the great infectious-disease scourges. Mortality rates from pneumococcal pneumonia were greater than 30 percent. By the late 1940s antibiotics seemed to have solved the problem, with mortality dropping to about 5 percent. Effective vaccine against common pneumococcal strains, however, has the distinct advantage of preventing rather than curing this serious infection, particularly in certain population subgroups.

In a study in the 1950s, Austrian demonstrated the continued prevalence of pneumococcal pneumonia. Austrian found through studies that two-thirds of patients with bacteremia (spillover of pneumococci into the bloodstream) who died were irreversibly injured during the first five days of infection, regardless of the therapy used. For these patients, prevention was the only solution. Moreover, the diagnosis of the cause of pneumonia can be difficult. In patients with bacteremia, the causative organism can be readily determined through simple blood cultures. In contrast, pneumococcal infections without bacteremia, accounting for 80 percent of the total, are difficult to diagnose. For these patients, precise diagnosis would require use of invasive techniques that are ethically not considered worth the small but finite risk to most patients.

The pneumococcal vaccine developed by Austrian, which in its latest form is actually like twenty-three vaccines in one (corresponding to the twenty-three most prevalent pneumococcal strains) was found in initial studies to provide a 78 percent reduction in proved or putative pneumococcal infections, and an 82 percent reduction in bacteremic infection—conclusive evidence of the vaccine's effectiveness. FDA approved the vaccine, it was marketed by Merck, and it became the first one ever covered by Medicare. Physician acceptance has been slow, however, for a number of reasons. First, the pneumococcal vaccine was marketed right after the swine flu episode. This did little to generate enthusiasm for a new vaccine. Second, most physicians do not appear to believe pneumococcal infection is much of a problem (fewer than 5 percent of hospitals routinely do the bacteriologic test required to identify pneumococci accurately). Third, internists are not attuned to giving vaccines, which is typically the province of pediatricians. Finally, the CDC's Advisory Committee on Immunization Practices gave the pneumococcal vaccine only a lukewarm recommendation, based on its assessment, which, according to an editorial by Austrian, was itself based on a flawed analysis by the Centers for Disease Control.

CDC's study included some children under ten years of age, who may be unable to mount or sustain a response to the vaccine. It also included certain adults whose immune systems were already compromised by therapy they were receiving for Hodgkins disease or leukemia.

Austrian concluded that—given these limitations in the CDC analysis design—the CDC data presented strongly suggest the utility of pneumococcal vaccine for immunocompetent persons over ten years of age who are at high risk of death from infection with this organism. He further concluded that the data provide a basis for wider physician acceptance and for continued CDC monitoring of the vaccine's efficacy.[60]

Merck, surprised by the inertia of physicians in vaccinating patients, broke with tradition and began using newspaper and magazine ads to consumers, suggesting they ask their physician's advice on whether or not to be vaccinated. This is one of the first instances of advertising directly to consumers since the 1938 Food, Drug and Cosmetic Act ushered in the widespread marketing of prescription drugs and advertising aimed at physicians. The reaction of patients and physicians is being watched with interest by the industry.

Finally, since the vaccine is relatively costly at about $1 per inoculation, its acceptance in developing nations, where pneumococcal pneumonia is still a major killer, has been slow.

The Guardian's Early Responses to Orphan Drugs

The FDA, though developing no specific policies, did begin to make individual provisions for review of certain orphan drugs brought to its attention by academic drug sponsors during the late 1960s and early 1970s. Additionally, according to Stuart Nightingale of the FDA, the agency's Bureau of Biologics considers the entire field of biologics to be an orphan-drug category, and has continued to help CDC and NIAID develop and make available new biologic products, including vaccines.[61]

Shortcuts to approval of orphan drugs, however, were ephemeral and not well known to drug manufacturers or academic drug sponsors. For instance, FDA officials commented at one meeting in 1977 that mechanisms existed for expediting review processes of drugs of limited commercial value; but, when asked for guidelines, FDA officials said they were informal and varied according to the situation.[62]

One special case has been identified in a report by an FDA review panel concerning approval of L-dopa for Parkinsons disease. It has an estimated U.S. prevalence of approximately 500,000. Because L-dopa was to be used on a long-term basis by patients, usually starting in the fourth or fifth decade of life, clinical safety tests could themselves take decades. Since therapeutic benefits were considered to outweigh by far potential risks, the FDA approved L-dopa for marketing on a gradual release basis with postmarket monitoring to be undertaken by the drug sponsor.[63]

Prior to FDA approval, the Parkinsons Disease Foundation reportedly spent $100,000 to purchase L-dopa from a foreign firm in order to have supplies for clinical studies in the United States. According to Roger Duvoisin of Rutgers, it was several years before clinical researchers were able to get the drug from U.S. firms. Duvoisin cited the drug's nonpatentable status (it is a normal constituent of the body) and its relatively limited market potential as barriers to industry interest in conducting clinical trials and marketing the drug here.[64]

The FDA Review Panel Report on New Drug Regulation also contained another recommendation especially applicable to orphan drugs, particularly those developed by academic scientists who had little experience developing protocols or data for FDA. The panel recommended that FDA increase its advisory committee use to review important INDs and provide expert assistance for developing protocols for promising new drugs, so as to avoid unnecessary delays later in the review process. The recommendation was intended for all promising new drugs; but, as former National Cancer Institute (NCI) director C. Gordon Zubrod commented, it was especially relevant for orphan drugs.

Zubrod said a special relationship existed between FDA and NCI from the late 1960s to the early 1970s, when FDA participated in NCI drug meetings and discussed data interpretation. FDA supervised NCI's drugs more through the spirit than by the letter of regulations. This cooperative approach, commended by Zubrod, gave way in the 1970s to uniformity in FDA's relationship with NCI and with industry, most often characterized as arm's length if not adversarial. Zubrod questioned whether the public good was best served this way, or by a regulatory policy that could speed up investigation of promising drugs while blocking unsafe and ineffective ones, whether developed within government, industry, or academia.[65]

FDA had recognized the particular problems attending anticancer drug development and had developed the Group C designation for drugs developed by the NCI. Along a similar line, FDA established the Compassionate IND or Treatment IND mechanism to make other drugs available before the review process had been completed for certain important drugs, including those distributed by CDC. In all these cases, physicians are required to provide information on the experimental use of the drug, and patients must sign consent forms. Physicians and drug developers were unfamiliar with these mechanisms, however, and no specific guidelines were in place. FDA's former director of the Bureau of Drugs, J. Richard Crout, speculated that physicians might not know of Compassionate INDs, and that FDA did not maintain a list in an organized way. He considered the process cumbersome and often unnecessary if drug sponsors instead would submit necessary data for approval of a new drug application.[66] Industry officials meanwhile commented that, because the process was unwieldy for them, they consented to participate only as a public service. The problem was acknowledged recently by Assistant Secretary for Health Brandt, who stated that an FDA committee currently is engaged in developing a systematic approach to Treatment and Compassionate INDs. This includes the process of designating appropriate drugs, publicizing their availability, and determining which drugs currently are available under this process.[67]

The FDA review panel also recommended that FDA be able to

require special studies for drugs being used widely for an unapproved purpose, where there is insufficient data to support safety and effectiveness of the drug for that use. The recommendation itself was not implemented; but, in the case of one orphan drug, ACTH, FDA did catalyze efforts to secure a supplemental NDA for its use in multiple sclerosis. The hormone, available from nineteen pharmaceutical firms, stimulates adrenal secretion of cortisone and had been found to shorten flare-up periods of multiple sclerosis symptoms. Multi-institutional clinical trials had been supported by the NINCDS, but the data never had been prepared for submission to FDA. Therefore, reimbursement for the drug—and, more important, for hospitalization needed for the drug's administration—was denied by third-party insurers. The FDA requested that the data be submitted in support of a supplemental NDA. A university researcher involved in the clinical trials volunteered to assemble and provide the data and shortly thereafter the supplemental NDA was approved.

As discussed in chapter 2, many drugs available for common diseases were not tested in rare conditions during development because firms feared any adverse effects related to the rare-disease use would hold up FDA approval of the drug for the common use. Therefore, the possibility that some marketed drugs might have additional orphan uses seems to be underexplored by industry.

A fourth issue raised by the FDA review panel pertaining to all drugs but especially significant for some orphan drugs is the degree to which FDA will accept foreign data in support of an NDA. This question is still under scrutiny at FDA. Industry is pressing for a policy of approval based on foreign studies. FDA cites problems in interpreting foreign data and in all but one instance has required foreign studies to be accompanied by two well-controlled U.S. studies. The issue is especially significant for orphan drugs, many of which appear to be available in Europe prior to marketing in this country. This may be due in part to industry's willingness to test drugs for small markets in countries where premarket testing expenses are not as high, where regulatory review may be faster, and where diseases that are rare in the United States may be more prevalent.

In the case of sodium valproate for epilepsy, for instance, ten years of successful marketing in Europe did not meet FDA criteria for U.S. approval. In the mid-1970s FDA had announced that foreign data would be accepted, but only when accompanied by two U.S. studies. In response, NINCDS supported and helped conduct two trials of sodium valproate for use in certain generalized seizure disorders. Thereafter, pressure was applied by interested physicians and patients and by the Epilepsy Foundation of America to induce Abbott to submit the NDA to FDA. Although approval was forthcoming, it required this type of major effort even though the drug was known to be an effective anticonvulsant and had been in widespread use for a decade elsewhere. FDA's foreign data requirements are not clear, although the agency recently did approve one drug primarily on the basis of foreign data.

According to Richard Crout, FDA has compiled available literature on certain drugs and has sought sponsors for drugs both before and after approving an NDA. He cited as examples potassium perchlorate for thyroid gland protection against radiation during brain scans, potassium iodide for thyroid protection against radiation from a nuclear reactor disaster, and THC (marijuana's active ingredient) for nausea and vomiting resulting from anticancer drugs. Additionally, Crout described efforts by FDA staff to meet with clinical investigators using orphan drugs experimentally in order to assist them in designing studies commensurate with NDA application requirements. FDA also has arranged for animal safety tests for some of these drugs to be performed by NCI or by the National Center for Toxicological Research.[68]

The era of patchwork policy had witnessed many successes. It had helped to define the range of issues faced, to promote specific programs, to facilitate review and approval of isolated orphan-drug cases, to provide access to certain unmarketed (Compassionate IND) drugs, and to assure redress for adverse effects from one vaccine program.

By the mid- to late 1970s, however, FDA determined that a more systematic approach was needed. The agency became the motivating force in establishing two interagency task forces to look into problems of orphan drugs, assess needs, and propose solutions. The first was convened in 1975 and the second in 1978. As will be developed in chapter 5, these were the first systematic efforts to come to grips with issues posed by orphan drugs. The task forces came at a time when the regulatory process itself was under critical review, and when issues pertaining to review and approval of all drugs were becoming both better defined and more worrisome. Issues of patent protection, liability, availability in the United States of drugs marketed abroad, and increased R&D costs all were becoming subjects of concern. To industry, orphan drugs represented extreme amplifications of all these problems.

The task forces also came at time when the scientific basis of drug discovery was undergoing a momentous shift due to newly emerging cell-biology techniques. As Crout commented, although progress on orphan drugs was being made, FDA anticipated that sophisticated modern biomedical research would present increasing numbers of orphan-drug candidates. He cited as examples possible cell-biology research on rare genetic, metabolic, or endocrine diseases; neurological disorders; and cancers. He warned that government should anticipate this trend and implement federal processes adequate to bring these new discoveries rapidly to fruition.

Academic orphan-drug researchers, like those involved in studies pertaining to drugs for more common diseases, were caught unprepared in this environment of rapidly changing technologies and of new university-industry arrangements. Whether orphan drugs were to lose even this shaky home was no longer merely an academic question.

Notes

1. James H. Young, "Public Policy and Drug Innovation," *Pharmacy in History*, 24(1) (1982).

2. E. Redman, *The Dance of Legislation* (New York: Simon and Schuster, 1973).

3. Edward Burger, "The Current Role of the Federal Government in Drug-Related R&D: What Is It and What Should It Be?" in S. Mitchell and E. Link, eds., *The Impact of Public Policy on Drug Innovation and Pricing* (Washington D.C.: American Unviersity, 1976).

4. Vincent DeVita, V.T. Oliverio, F.M. Muggia, P.W. Wiernik, J. Ziegler, A. Goldin, D. Rubin, J. Henney, S. Schepartz. "The Drug Development and Clinical Trials Programs of the Division of Cancer Treatment, National Cancer Institute," *Cancer Clinical Trials* 2(1979):195–216.

5. C.G. Zubrod, S. Schepartz, J. Leiten, K.M. Endicott, L.M. Carrese, C.E. Baker, *Cancer Chemotherapy Reports: October 1966* 50(7)(Bethesda, Md.: U.S. DHEW, 1968).

6. DeVita et al., "Drug Development," p. 205.

7. Ibid., p. 204.

8. Saul Schepartz, NCI, personal communication, 1981.

9. DeVita et al., "Drug Development," pp. 207–208.

10. William Hubbard, "Testimony Before the Subcommittee on Health and the Environment," U.S. House, Committee on Energy and Commerce, Congressman Henry A. Waxman, chairman, March 9, 1981.

11. "Rate of Development of Anticancer Drugs by the National Cancer Institute and the U.S. Pharmaceutical Industry and the Impact of Regulation," Final Report for the National Cancer Institute (New York: University of Rochester Medical Center, 1981), pp. ii, 40.

12. D. Mullally, NIAID, personal communication, 1980.

13. R.A. Krall et al., "Anti-epileptic Drug Development. I. History and a Program for Progress," *Epilepsia* 19(4)(1978):393–408.

14. National Institute of Neurological and Communicative Disorders and Stroke Antiepileptic Drug Development Program, *Program Performance Summary*, NINCDS, 1982.

15. Philip J. Hilts, "FDA Consultant Assails Upjohn's Lack of Contraceptive Studies," *Washington Post*, January 12, 1983.

16. *NHLBI Fact Book for Fiscal Year 1978* (Washington, D.C.: DHEW, 1979) pp. 79–99.

17. G.B. Kolata, "Drug Found to Help Heart Attack Survivors: An NHLBI Study of Propranolol," *Science* 214(1981):774–775.

18. Jack Anderson, "Drug Addicts: Unwilling Guinea Pigs," *Washington Post*, July 1, 1978, p. D15.

19. Stuart Nightingale, presentation to PMA Commission on Drugs for Rare Diseases, 1982.

20. Roy Widdus, director, National Academy of Sciences Study on Private Sector Initiatives in Vaccines, personal communication, June 1984.

21. Office of Technology Assessment, *A Review of Selected Federal Vaccine and Immunization Policies* PB80-116106 (Washington, D.C.: NTIS, September 1979).

22. David Schwartzman, *Innovation in the Pharmaceutical Industry* (Baltimore, Md.: Johns Hopkins University Press, 1976), p. 19.

23. Milton Silverman and Philip R. Lee, *Pills, Profits and Politics* (Berkeley: University of California Press, 1974), p. 236.

24. Sandra Ford, "Drugs for Parasitic Diseases," in Fred E. Karch, ed., *Orphan Drugs* (New York: Marcel Dekker, 1982), pp. 168–180.

25. R. Hopkins, in appendix to Interim Report of the Committee on Drugs of Limited Commercial Value (Rockville, Md.: FDA, 1975).

26. William Haddad, GPIA president, personal communication, 1984.

27. Walter Dowdle, "Statement of Walter Dowdle, Ph.D., Director, Center for Infectious Diseases, Centers for Disease Control," in *Cost Effectiveness of the Influenza Vaccine*, February 5, 1982, in *Health and the Environment Miscellaneous*, Part 7, Serial No. 97-128 (Washington, D.C.: U.S. Government Printing Office, 1982), p. 106.

28. Dowdle, "Statement," p. 124.

29. Frederick C. Robbins, "Statement of Frederick C. Robbins, M.D., President, Institute of Medicine, National Academy of Sciences," in *Childhood Immunizations*, February 4, 1982, Ibid., p. 8.

30. James Chin, "Statement of James Chin, M.D., Infectious Disease Section, California Department of Health Services," Ibid., p. 33.

31. Chin, "Statement," p. 34.

32. Tim Westmoreland, Ibid., p. 26.

33. David Banta and Jane Sisk, "Statement of David Banta, Assistant Director for Health and Life Sciences, and Jane Sisk, Ph.D., Project Director, Office of Technology Assessment," Ibid., p. 46.

34. Office of Technology Assessment, *Cost Effectiveness of Influenza*

Vaccination (Washington, D.C.: Congress of the United States, December 1981), p. 6.

35. Dowdle, *Cost Effectiveness of the Influenza Vaccine*, p. 103.

36. Ibid., p. 107.

37. Milton Silverman, Philip R. Lee, and Mia Lydecker, *Prescriptions for Death: The Drugging of the Third World* (Berkeley: Unviersity of California Press, 1982).

38. Myron Schultz, "Current Concepts in Parasitology," *New England Journal of Medicine* 297(1977):1259.

39. Proceedings Summary, "Need for New Drug Development: Problems in Reorienting Drug Research," *WHO Chronicle* 32(4)(1978):154–155.

40. Richard Neustadt and Harvey Fineberg, *The Swine Flu Affair: Decision-Making on a Slippery Disease*, No. 017-000-00210-4 (Washington, D.C.: U.S. Government Printing Office, 1978), pp. 48–63.

41. Jane S. Willems, "Statement of Jane Willems, Ph.D., Project Director, Office of Technology Assessment," *Cost-Effectiveness of the Influenza Vaccine*, p. 71.

42. Dowdle, "Statement," pp. 113–114.

43. Henry Grabowski, J. Vernon, and L. Thomas, "The Effects of Regulatory Policy on the Incentives to Innovate: An International Comparative Analysis," in S. Mitchell and E. Link, eds., *The Impact of Public Policy in Drug Innovation and Pricing* (Washington, D.C.: American University, 1976), pp. 47–82.

44. Neil Nathanson and A.D. Langmuir, "The Cutter Incident. Poliomyelitis Following Vaccination in the United States During the Spring of 1955," *American Journal of Hygiene* 78(1963):16–81.

45. Frederick Robbins, "Statement," *Childhood Immunizations*, pp. 9–10.

46. Cristine Russell, "Maker of Vaccine Quits Over Liability," *Washington Post*, June 19, 1984.

47. Neustadt and Fineberg, *Swine Flu Affair*, pp. 49–52.

48. Neustadt and Fineberg, Ibid. pp. 48–62.

49. A.K. Asbury, personal communication, May 17, 1984.

50. Lawrence B. Schonberger, E.S. Hurwitz, P. Katona, R.C. Holman, and D.J. Bregman, "Guillain-Barre Syndrome: Its Epidemiology and Associations with Influenza Vaccination," *Annals of Neurology* 9(1981)(suppl.):31–38.

51. A.K. Asbury, "Diagnostic Considerations in Guillain-Barre Syndrome," *Annals of Neurology* 9(suppl)(1981):1–5.

52. A.K. Asbury, personal communication.

53. Associated Press, "Parents in Vaccine Deaths Ask Compensation Surcharge," *Philadelphia Inquirer*, May 4, 1984, p. A13.

54. Grabowski, Vernon, and Thomas, "Effects of Regulatory Policy."

55. FTC Reports, March 6, 1984, p. 17, and correction printed April 9, 1984, p. 11 ("In Brief").

56. Edwin Chen, "Liability Suits: Few Guidelines," *L.A. Times*, October 6, 1982.

57. Marlene Cimons, "Women's Group to Sue Maker of Contraceptive," *L.A. Times*, January 11, 1983.

58. Chen, "Liability Suits."

59. Robert Temple, Presentation at Physicians Responsibility in Medicine and Research Meeting, Philadelphia, April 1984.

60. Robert Austrian, "The Assessment of Pneumococcal Vaccine," *New England Journal of Medicine* 303(1980):578–580.

61. Stuart Nightingale, "Presentation to the PMA Commission on Drugs for Rare Diseases," February 18, 1982, p. 3.

62. C.H. Asbury, "Medical Drugs of Limited Commercial Interest: The Development of Federal Policy," Masters thesis, Johns Hopkins University School of Hygiene and Public Health, 1981, p. 48.

63.. Review Panel on New Drug Regulation (Washington D.C.: DHEW, May 1977).

64. Roger Duvoisin, Statement before the Subcommittee on Health and the Environment, Committee on Energy and Commerce, March 8, 1982.

65. Zubrod, *Cancer Chemotherapy Reports*.

66. J. Richard Crout, Jr., Statement before the Subcommittee on Health and the Environment, March 9, 1981, p. 7.

67. Edward Brandt, Jr., Statement before the Subcommittee on Health and the Environment, March 8, 1982, p. 8.

68. Crout, "Statement," pp. 4–7.

4
A New Era in Patents, Publishing, and Policy

J ust as chemical technologies developed by industry ushered in the era of antibiotic wonder drugs and prompted firms to integrate vertically to control patent profits, so today are university-developed molecular-biology techniques inspiring new forms of horizontal coordination between industry and academia.

Although university-based cell biology may be supplanting chemistry as the basis for some important new therapeutic advances, industry still has the means to realize the clinical applications of these advances by conducting large-scale trials, preparing NDAs, and marketing and distributing products. In the emerging horizontal coordination of university and industry R&D, industry pressures to maintain patent rights and trade-secret status of data may clash with university pressures to publish research results. In some cases, questions of conflict of interest are attracting as much attention as the research itself. Yet the potential for major new discoveries exists.

At no time has it been more complicated to establish patent, royalty, and licensing rights than in today's turbulent environment of joint ventures; spinoff companies; cooperative, collaborative, or contractual R&D arrangements; affiliate programs; or information exchange activities. Making patent assessments even more difficult is the continuing involvement of federal funds, either indirectly, through research grants, or directly, through federal joint-venture participation.

Accompanying these uncertainties are worries about whether industry funding of academic research will halt early dissemination of scientific findings through journal publications and scientific meetings, constrained by the need to preserve not only patents but also the trade-secret status of data.

Industry funding will have both anticipated and unexpected consequences. Some academic-based orphan-drug researchers question whether these new joint arrangements will propel university research in new directions—for instance, toward applied instead of basic research, and away from R&D on orphan drugs toward development of more commonly used products.

The situation calls for action as opposed to reaction. Will the development of new therapies entail an *and* or an *or* relationship with the development of commercially profitable products.

Current Types of Arrangements

Several large-scale arrangements for long-term university-industry research ventures have arisen in the past few years. Among these are Harvard-Monsanto, Harvard Medical School–Seagrams, Massachusetts General Hospital–Hoechst, Washington University–Mallinckrodt Inc., Washington University–Monsanto, MIT-Exxon, and Carnegie Mellon–Westinghouse, according to a recent National Science Foundation (NSF) report.[1]

Additionally, as NSF points out, there has been a spate of new biotechnology firms. In 1978, for instance, there were four companies worldwide that specialized in industrial applications of recombinant-DNA technologies. By 1981 there were about 110 such firms, and total capitalization had increased from $20 million for the original four companies to about $700 million. NSF reports an additional 70 firms are working on monoclonal antibody research. Many of these apparently have academic advisors or consultants; others are spinoff companies founded and owned by academic scientists.

NSF concludes that only larger industrial companies form industry-university arrangements; smaller companies interact more informally through knowledge transfer programs of various types. NSF uses specific criteria to categorize these arrangements. *Resources* refer to gifts in support of university research, highly valued because they are flexible and provide benefits that exceed the dollar value of support. Gifts, however, do not necessarily promote interaction between donor and recipient. *Cooperative research* refers to informal scientific interaction in planning general approaches to research and its applications. This is achieved by: (1) contracts between individual investigators and corporations; (2) industrial-affiliates programs, whereby members of companies bring technical problems of a nonproprietary nature to faculty and students; and (3) provision of institutional facilities, such as research centers, that attract industry support by providing a central place for equipment, research coordination, and focus. These approaches, now more common than ever before, date back to the early 1900s.

Historical Cooperative Precedents

Joint ventures between academic scientists and major R&D companies, which today receive a great deal of media attention in the fields of biotechnology and pharmaceuticals, were used in the disciplines of engineering and physics shortly after the turn of the century, as described in the NSF report.[2]

Between 1910 and 1930, industrial and university research laboratories flourished, the latter's programs funded largely through philanthropic gifts from private individuals, corporations, and large foundations. Specific examples illustrate the three general types of cooperative arrangements at that time. From 1913 to 1930, MIT's Research Laboratory for Applied Chemistry attracted financial support from companies seeking answers to specific chemical problems. Meanwhile, Cal Tech had established a cooperative research program on fundamental scientific issues of interest to private industry, funded by industrial and foundation philanthropy. Cal Tech also had a major aerospace program under a long-term grant from the David Guggenheim Fund. The University of Illinois established a rich industrial network connection for its Ph.D.s involved in commercial manufacture of rare organic chemicals. Industry helped finance two chemical journals founded by the unviersity, as well as consultantships and fellowships for graduate students.

This close industrial-academic cooperation was strengthened during the war years but deteriorated during the 1950s and 1960s as federal research funding increased. Since then, industry has supported about 3 percent to 4 percent of the total academic research allocations. About one-half of this support has been in the field of engineering. Constant dollars have increased, but the percentage has remained relatively stable. If corporate philanthropic support is included in the percentage of research funding, however, the figure may be as high as 6 percent to 7 percent of academic R&D, representing between $400 and $450 million.

Early Pharmaceutical Cooperation

Between the 1930s and the 1950s, pharmaceuticals began to be part of this cooperative approach between industry and academia. Three of the best-known examples, as discussed by Schwartzman, concern types of orphan drugs: the polio vaccine, birth control pills, and unpatentable corticosteroids. In each of these instances, joint participation was facilitated by voluntary health organizations, which continue to this day to play a major role in support of orphan-drug development.

The polio vaccine primarily demonstrates cooperation between academic and voluntary health groups. Jonas Salk's University of Pittsburgh laboratory was supported in large measure by the National Foundation for Infantile Paralysis, whose research director, Harry Weaver, convinced Salk and his associates to mount an intensive investigation into the possibility of developing a polio vaccine. At the same time, according to Schwartzman, that other researchers were ruling out the vaccination approach, the Salk team was conducting a virus-typing program developed by Weaver, whose optimism for development of a successful vaccine had been fueled by prior findings by other scientists funded by the foundation. Among these were the demonstration by John Enders at Harvard that virus could be grown in tissues other than those of the nervous system, dispelling the theory that polio virus could be grown only in living nerve cells. Additionally, Isabel Mountain had reported that polio virus inactivated with formalin produced antibody and immunity at levels similar to that of live virus, introducing the possibility that an effective killed-virus vaccine could be developed. Massive infusion of dollars from the foundation and solid scientific leads provided Salk with the means to develop one of the most heralded public-health benefits of modern time.

In the case of cortisone, an unpatentable natural adrenal hormone discussed at length in chapter 2, initial development was expedited by cooperation between Merck and the Mayo Clinic scientists, with additional efforts by several other universities and by Squibb, according to Schwartzman's account. The National Research Council served as catalyst in wartime 1942 by authorizing development of the chemical technology required to synthesize enough corticosteroids to study cortisone's activity, based on a preliminary indication that the drug would be an important therapeutic advance in treating a number of conditions.

The first birth control pill marketed here, the third example, emerged from research conducted at the Worcester Foundation for Biological Research, a nonprofit private laboratory; the research had been urged by the Planned Parenthood Foundation. Based on a prior finding by academic scientists that rabbits injected with progesterone did not ovulate, Worcester's Gregory Pincus found the same effect could be achieved with orally administered progesterone. Small-scale clinical trials then were conducted in collaboration with John Rock of Harvard.

These initial clinical trials revealed that high oral doses were required, prompting Pincus to seek assistance from G.D. Searle Company. Searle's Frank Colton produced a norethynodrel, which was found by the Pincus-Rock team to be far more potent orally than progesterone. Here was a drug that was effective at a low dose, hence with little toxicity. Searle conducted large-scale clinical trials in Puerto Rico and received FDA approval to market the contraceptive in 1960.[3]

These successful examples of the 1950s involved problems similar to those confronting orphan-drug development today, notably lack of patent protection and high liability risks. Perhaps the large market potential and likelihood of major clinical advances outweighed those problems. Nonetheless, these past experiences of joint cooperation stand in sharp contrast to some of those recounted recently by academic scientists involved in drug development efforts.

University-Developed Orphan Drugs: Patent and Liability Issues

Many university-based orphan-drug examples of recent years are described in detail in the recent monograph edited by Fred Karch.[4] Clearly, one of the most prevalent themes was the difficulty in finding commercial sponsors for drugs that are not eligible for product patents, as was the case for five of the six drugs described. Only one of the unpatentable drugs, dopamine, eventually was conjointly developed by industry and academia—by researchers at Emory University and Arnar-Stone Laboratories (a division of American Hospital Supply Corporation)—and marketed as a pressor agent for use in treating shock and congestive heart failure.[5]

Many of the unpatented drugs brought to light in the Karch edition and through other discussions had other, confounding problems. For instance, two academic-based drug developers encountered insurmountable obstacles to obtaining liability coverage through their universities. One of these researchers had developed and secured an NDA on an unpatentable diagnostic radiological dye after several drug companies he contacted said the product was not of sufficient economic interest. FDA had requested he submit the NDA so that FDA reviewers would not have to approve each individual IND submitted by radiologists seeking permission to use the diagnostic product. The NDA actually was awarded to the nonprofit institution that employed the researcher, but the institution refused to make the dye available commercially because the cost of obtaining liability insurance was prohibitive. The university signed the patent over to the researcher, who, with venture capital, sought to create a firm to market the product.[6]

A second example of liability insurance problems concerns aceto-hydroxamic acid, developed by Donald Griffith at Baylor University, for dissolving infection-induced urinary stones. This condition is particularly problematic for paraplegics or quadraplegics, a group that includes a number of returning Vietnam veterans. Because the drug was a shelf chemical, it was not eligible for a product patent. Patients were relatively few and widely scattered; most had other medical problems, making it difficult to conduct and coordinate clinical trials. Attempts to secure liability insurance, exacerbated by a laboratory accident, compounded the problem. Baylor officials refused to buy insurance, considering it astronomically costly, and in its absence decided it was unwise to prepare and distribute the drug for use in other institutions where researchers were participating in the study. Even Baylor's continued involvement with the drug was curtailed because of these product liability constraints. Griffith, having approached forty pharmaceutical firms unsuccessfully, finally formed a small corporation with venture capital to prepare the NDA application.[7]

A third example of liability problems plus lack of patent protection comes from British researcher John Walshe.[8] He initially developed penicillamine, a lifesaving drug for the few thousand patients with Wilsons disease, a disorder of copper metabolism. In Wilsons disease victims, copper is deposited in the liver, causing cirrhosis, and in the brain, causing damage in regions controlling movement. If not treated by the chelating agent penicillamine (a metabolite of penicillin), patients die of liver failure or neurological deterioration and terminal infection within a few years. One need only read Berton Roueché's moving article in the *New Yorker* to grasp the extraordinary problems patients face, both in obtaining correct diagnosis of the disorder and in coping with its effects without treatment until the diagnosis is made.[9] Penicillamine was developed by Walshe and approved by the FDA for use in Wilsons disease prior to the 1962 FDA amendments. In those days, Walshe says, clinical trials were simple. He obtained penicillamine from a scientist at MIT, and both he and a patient took the drug. Neither suffered ill effects, and both excreted a large amount of copper. Back in England, Walshe found a commercial source for the chemical and conducted initial therapeutic trials. Eventually the drug, sponsored by Merck in the United States, was approved by FDA.

Some time later, however, Walshe found some patients were not able to tolerate penicillamine; they developed allergic reactions to it. He sought a substitute in the form of trien (triethylene tetramine dihydrochloride). This was a crude industrial chemical, an oily, corrosive, strongly alkaline liquid used as an epoxy resin hardener. Walshe prepared trien, purified it, and packed it by hand into capsules for a few patients who needed to take it. When initial supplies were found to have a toxic impurity, a meeting was held with representatives from industry and from malpractice insurance societies, doctors, a medical ethicist, and some journalists. Fear of litigation was found to be the major problem; companies feared damage suits and loss of good name.

Walshe writes that the Laboratory of the Government Chemist agreed to test the final product as well as the source material for purity. Walshe then could secure a product license, provided he give written acceptance of full responsibility for all possible consequences. But the Department of Health did not take out the product license. Instead, it requested that Walshe produce protocols for clinical testing of the drug over a ten-year period, in which three new patients per year were to be added. At the time of publication of Karch's book, Walshe reported that with an increase in the number of patients needing trien to nineteen, the requests for his homemade medication reached 2,000 capsules per month. Finally, the Laboratory of the Government Chemist laid down specifications for purity, and Cambrian Chemical began manufacturing the drug to these specifications.

Liability coverage was not a major factor for the drug L-5HTP, used in postanoxic myoclonus and developed by Melvin Van Woert at Mount Sinai Hospital and Medical Center in New York. In this case, however, the combination of small market potential and unpatentability of the shelf chemical proved to be solid barriers to commercial involvement. Van Woert explains that he purchased the chemical in powder form from Calbiochem, a San Diego firm, for $2,200 per kilogram, an average of $135 per month per patient. An NIH grant covered animal studies and purchase of the drug for short-term therapeutic trials, but not for long-term therapeutic and clinical pharmacologic investigation. An increase in the number of patients and the need for the clinical investigators to encapsulate the drug themselves forced Van Woert to seek alternative means for continuing the work. The National Myoclonus Foundation was established by dedicated volunteers who provided some interim support through vigorous fund-raising efforts. Van Woert sought assistance from NIH, FDA, various pharmaceutical companies, and finally legislators (chapter 5). All were sympathetic to the problem, but none were able to provide solutions.[10]

The critical role of patents in transferring university-developed inventions into the marketplace is evidenced by activities of the Research Corporation, a nonprofit foundation for the advancement of science and technology. For new inventions, the corporation acts as an intermediary between researchers (whether from universities or from other nonprofit institutions) and potential industrial sponsors. Through agreements with nearly 300 nonprofit educational and scientific institutions, the foundation accepts assignment of certain inventions. It evaluates the invention's likely scientific or technical merits, patentability, and commercial potential.

For inventions selected by these criteria, the corporation donates its services in seeking patents and potential licensees. Royalties from successfully licensed inventions are distributed between the inventor's institution and the Research Corporation in percentages previously agreed on. Inventors usually are assigned a percentage of gross royalties, determined by their institution's policies, with the remainder divided equally by the institution and the Research Corporation. The corporation uses its share to support basic research in the natural and physical sciences through grants to nonprofit institutions. In its brochures, the corporation emphasizes that many manufacturers are unwilling to invest in new technologies that are not patent protected. Because almost any invention can be awarded some type of patent, emphasis is placed on inventions likely to be awarded a patent that is broad enough to support a licensing program; this generally means a product patent.[11]

Corporation brochures also emphasize that its lawyers should evaluate the invention before any reseach data are published. This advice stems from a U.S. patent law provision that applications must be filed within one year after data publication. Foreign patents are even more constraining: They will not be granted once data are published, and there is no grace period.

These patent restrictions on data publication are at odds with demands of university tenure committees and federal granting agencies to "publish or perish" or "publish, period," respectively. This double bind, which exists for academic drug developers in general, is illuminated by tales from a few of the orphan-drug sponsors writing in the Karch edition.

Patent or Publish? Some Orphan Examples

The first case concerns dopamine, mentioned earlier. Emory University scientists developed the drug for use in shock and congestive heart failure. Emory officials, aware that the drug was not eligible for a product patent because dopamine is a natural substance, wanted to apply for a use patent in the hope of attracting a commercial sponsor; they requested permission from NIH officials to do so. NIH officials pressed instead for prompt publication of dopamine data. Only later, according to dopamine developer Leon Goldberg, did the scientists learn they actually had a choice in the matter; only later did they find out they might have had a chance to secure a foreign patent if they had not published their data beforehand. Nonetheless, the dopamine incident had a happy ending. John Zaroslinski of Arnar-Stone Laboratories already had a interest in what he and the firm determined was an important medical product. Because the intended market size was anticipated to be relatively small and thus not likely to entice generic manufacturers, the firm developed the drug conjointly with Emory University and marketed dopamine in the absence of patent protection.

Other drug candidates did not fare as well. Stephen De Felice of Bio/Basics International encountered a number of problems in developing the natural substance carnitine for several potential uses. In an unconventional approach, De Felice initiated acute animal toxicity studies but also began phase I clinical testing abroad, using intravenous carnitine. Two colleagues took large doses of the drug themselves to try to establish appropriate dosage levels, but this produced transient illnesses in the investigators. Once the studies got back on the track, De Felice did not publish data on carnitine for fear of jeopardizing possible patent opportunities. By not publishing, De Felice concluded, he may have made academic clinical researchers leery of becoming involved in drug trials. Carnitine, again a natural substance, might have been eligible for use patents. Because the drug had several potential clinical applications, however, use patents would be difficult to enforce. As De Felice mused, imagine if carnitine were a simple substance, with a single indication and strong patent position: Carnitine long ago would have been marketed, and his life would be less difficult and more secure.[12] Much went wrong with this drug case, but it illustrates the dilemma investigators face when they try to gain scientific acceptance while maintaining proprietary options.

With the new surge of industry-university joint ventures, maintaining scientific communication while not compromising proprietary position is an increasingly major problem. Even if scientists are allowed one year from the time of publication to file a U.S. patent claim, this can be tricky, not to mention its implications for loss of foreign patents.

Another illustrative orphan-drug case is told by James Stubbins of the Medical College of Virginia. While funded on an NIH grant, Stubbins began development of a long-acting topical anesthetic. The product was patentable (the only patentable product among the six described in the Karch edition). Stubbins published his data, reassured by his knowledge that he had a year therafter to file for a patent claim. He filed the claim in November 1967. Unbeknownst to him, however, a Swedish firm also had developed a similar long-acting topical anesthetic. The Swedish firm's product contained some of the same atoms as Stubbin's compound, but the concept for achieving long duration of action differed. The resulting interference conference convened by the U.S. Patent and Trademark Office produced a decision in favor of the Swedish firm. The decision was based on the finding that Stubbins had not acted "diligently" in translating the discovery into practice following receipt of the NIH grant. After Stubbins amended his claim, it was disallowed because it encompassed more than one structural type. Resubmission of the two new patent claims, one for each structural type, occurred more than one year after Stubbin's initial publication: By then the data were in the public domain. Stubbins, meanwhile, was out a patent—or perhaps two.[13]

A Broader Perspective on the Issues

Patent and trade-secret status of data protection are now prime concerns for universities and their scientists. Federal granting agencies' patent policies, confusing at best, have come under heavy criticism.[14] In 1980, Congress enacted the Uniform Federal Patent Policy Act (P.L. 96-517) to permit universities, nonprofit firms, and small businesses to take title to inventions resulting from federally funded R&D.[15] NIH's Leroy Randall has said this law basically codified NIH patent policies that have been in use by the agency for the past twenty years. Universities now submit uniform patent forms.

According to Randall, university scientists are asked to estimate the potential development costs and demonstrate how the public might benefit from the invention. On the basis of this information, the DHHS secretary signs a waiver determination, which in effect signs the patent over to the university. As a rule, the university patent holder can be expected to find commercial licensees who in turn will generate royalties back to the university. If university officials decide not to develop the invention, the university can return the patent. With P.L. 96-517, the university will have to pay a maintenance fee on each patent it retains every 3.6, 7.6, and 11.6 years after the patent is granted; fees go to support the U.S. Patent and Trademark Office. If fees are not paid, the patent will not be enforced. In addition, NIH (or any federal granting agency) has "march-in rights," whereby it can repossess the patent if the university does not develop an invention deemed important to the public welfare.

Currently NIH has no easily accessible record of how many federally funded inventions have resulted in products available to the public; it also has no lists or numbers of total patents NIH holds or of total patents that have been assigned to universities. The agency is in the process of setting up a computerized system for retrieving this type of information. According to Randall, the number of patents taken out by NIH has remained relatively constant on average during the past ten years. NIH receives about 600 invention reports per year. Of these, about 150 are on inventions developed by intramural (NIH) scientists or are patents rejected by universities. NIH seeks patents for about 50 of these inventions annually.[16] An aide to Senator Robert Dole (R-Kan.) reportedly estimated that 90 percent of government-held patents are not developed.[17]

According to some university scientists cited in a recent *Science* article, NIH has appeared more concerned with timely dissemination of research findings than with preservation or maximization of patent opportunities for NIH grantees. During the past few years, the Office of Management and Budget (OMB) has been taking steps to provide new regulations conferring greater uniformity in federal patent policies. Nonetheless, NIH continues to require that grantees inform the agency of every potentially patentable invention that may result from the grant. Critics have asserted that often scientists do not understand the details of the NIH requirements. Industry also is concerned, especially about NIH march-in rights provided in the 1980 Uniform Federal Patent Policy Act. What if, for instance, the government marches in to reclaim patent rights to a product for which industry supported prior research leading to the product?[18] Additionally, industry is concerned that publication of data funded by NIH—but also funded concurrently, or previously, by industry—might jeopardize patent claims.

One example that spins a web of these interrelated patent questions should illustrate the potential entanglements. It concerns a possible new and lucrative method for producing synthetic vaccines that may be safer than traditional attenuated live- or killed-virus vaccine. Trouble erupted with the almost simultaneous publication of articles on the new technique by two different research teams— one at the University of California, San Diego (UCSD), in collaboration with the Salk Institute, and the other at the nearby Scripps Clinic and Research Foundation at La Jolla. The UCSD/Salk team had submitted their manuscript for publication five days before the Scripps team did, but the Scripps group was the first to file a patent application.

Scripps had entered into a joint venture to produce the synthetic vaccines with Johnson & Johnson for an undisclosed sum, including funds for a new research building. A UCSD/Salk team scientist had discussed his team's work with a Scripps team scientist, who later told a member of the UCSD/Salk team that the Scripps group was doing the same type of research. The telchnology involved in identifying proteins immunologically and then causing antibodies to be produced against the protein or virus is a powerful tool for identifying viral proteins. The synthetic vaccine, like vaccines currently used, would stimulate antibody production against a specific virus. But whereas current vaccines use whole virus, synthetic vaccines would contain only the viral antigen (a specific protein). These proteins could be identified immunologically using rapid sequencing methods and then synthesized chemically. The new product thus would be expected to be purer and safer than traditional whole virus.

Beyond the question of who was first to devise the technique, there is the issue of whether scientific results should be placed first with the patent office or with the scientific community through journal articles. As the UCSD scientist put it, bad manners in science is one thing, but when you're talking big dollars, that uncorks a whole other matter.[19]

In still another example, NIH involvement complicated the picture. Scientists at UCLA, using funds from an NIH grant, successfully grew out in tissue culture a cell line from a patient with myelogenous leukemia. The cell line was called KG1. One of the UCLA scientists shared the line with an NIH scientist, who in turn discovered that the line produced low concentrations of interferon. This NIH scientist then sent some of the cells to a former NIH colleague now working on interferon research at the Roche Institute of Molecular Biology, a nonprofit research arm of Hoffmann-La-Roche. The Roche scientist transformed the KG1 line from a mild to a strong interferon-producing one. Thereupon Hoffmann-LaRoche, in collaboration with Genentech, applied for a patent. In a bitterly disputed case, UCLA scientists claimed the NIH scientist should not have shared the line with his Hoffmann-LaRoche colleague. As Barbara Culliton observes, amid suits and countersuits, the public and scientific communities witnessed a major fight between a drug house and a university, battling over the rightful ownership of cells initially developed with federal funding.[20]

As these two examples illustrate, patent ownership is becoming alarmingly complicated with the advent of cell biology technologies. These new techniques may produce hundreds of products, only some of which (or none) eventually may prove to be therapeutically useful. Moreover, it may become increasingly difficult to determine whether industry or government is the research sponsor of a particular product with the massive new infusion of industry funds expected in academic science.[21]

This expectation, based on the assumption that pharmaceutical firms are eager to help fund and retain future license or marketing rights to university-originated products, is bolstered further by a recently enacted law providing incentives to industry to support increased R&D. At about the time P.L. 96-517 became law in 1980, the Justice Department issued an "Antitrust Guide Concerning Research Joint Ventures," which sought to clarify conditions under which cooperative R&D ventures would be permissible under antitrust laws. The following year, the newly installed Reagan administration sought tax incentives for R&D investments by industry. The Economic Recovery Tax Act of 1981, P.L. 97-34, included: (1) a 25 percent tax credit for incremental R&D increases based on historic R&D expense levels; (2) a charitable-deduction increase (cost plus one-half the difference between cost and fair market value) for donated new equipment to an institution of higher education for research and training in physical and biological sciences; (3) a two-year suspension of tax regulations requiring allocation of research expenses between U.S. and foreign-source income, with further study of this by the Treasury Department; and (4) a three-year depreciation schedule on research equipment instead of the previous five-year stipulation.[22]

This came at a time when federal R&D funding had been steadily eroded for a decade by inflation and escalating university overhead, or indirect, costs. A 1984 General Accounting Office (GAO) report documents a staggering rise in indirect costs, claiming about 30 percent of NIH grant expenditures as of fiscal year (FY) 1982. According to the GAO study, university indirect-cost recovery rates have been subject to abrupt hikes, apparently to cover maintenance, administrators' salaries, and other operating expenses.[23] Meanwhile, funding directly to researchers, in constant dollars, has remained the same for the past ten years as inflation has eroded spending power. University administrators have countered by asserting that it is not a case of indirect costs rising disporportionately but rather of costs not being funded at levels commensurate with rises in inflation.[24]

A second factor that may enhance the environment for joint industry-university arrangements is the notable presence of important "boundary spanners"—primarily highly regarded academic scientists who recently have taken on major roles in pharmaceutical firms. For instance, Theodore Cooper—former NIH official, assistant secretary for health in the Ford administration, and former dean of Cornell Medical School—now is an executive vice-president at the Upjohn Company in Kalamazoo, Michigan. Notably, Cooper has been serving as the first chairman of the PMA's Commission on Drugs for Rare Diseases, to be discussed in later chapters. Charles Sanders recently left as director of the Massachusetts General Hospital (MGH) to become a vice-president at E.R. Squibb & Sons, Inc., of Princeton, New Jersey. P. Roy Vagelos moved from Washington University in St. Louis to become president of Merck, Sharp and Dohme Research Laboratories; W. Clark Wescoe, former chancellor of the University of Kansas, is now chairman of the board of Sterling Drug in New York.[25]

Universities are overhauling their patent postures to pave the way for favorable joint-venture arrangements. Changes in Harvard University's patent policy, for instance, have gained widespread attention as a bellwether, as traced by Barbara Culliton in a Distinguished Lectureship for Public Understanding of Science.[26] Initially the Harvard corporation required that any discoveries made in its laboratories be dedicated to the public, as explained by Bernard Davis.[27] This policy dates back to 1934, when the president and fellows of Harvard adopted a policy stipulating that no patents for therapeutic agents could be taken out by a faculty member except by University consent. In fact, legal advice would be provided to any university members desiring that steps be taken to prevent patenting by others. Finally, all patents that were taken out by the university would be dedicated to the public, according to Culliton.

By the mid-1970s, Harvard changed this policy. The university affirmed the guiding principle that public benefits should take precedence over making profits. Now, however, there was an emphasis on seeking patents aggressively. No longer was patent pursuit discouraged. Rather, faculty were to inform the university of any potentially patentable inventions or discoveries. This was similar to NIH policies put in place at about that time. The shift at Harvard took place at about the time the San Francisco-based biotechnology firm Genentech made its debut on Wall Street with opening-day stock prices that soared from their initial $35 per share offering to $89 per share. It also was about that time that Monsanto Chemical Corporation officials negotiated a $23 million collaboration with Harvard to extend over a ten-year period. Monsanto was interested primarily in research by a Harvard scientist working on the hypothesis that a particular factor (tumor angiogenesis factor) encouraged blood supply to tumors and therefore might show how to starve tumors by blocking its action. Monsanto agreed to fund the research, contribute endowment, and construct new laboratories in exchange for rights to the tumor-blocking agent if successfully developed. According to Culliton's analysis, the agreement was compromised because it was negotiated in secret and violated Harvard's long-held tradition of open communication. Terms were not revealed; no written evidence was presented of assurance that publication rights had been preserved. Moreover, there was no faculty involvement in proposing or negotiating terms.

Soon thereafter, Harvard's president, Derek Bok, proposed to the faculty that the university consider forming its own company. He outlined the pros and cons, and faculty members came up with some additional ones. Among problems cited were how to assure equal opportunity for publication, maintain priority of academic work, avoid conflict of interest, and preserve publishing rights and open discussion. Faculty judged the cons outweighed the pros, and the measure was rejected.

The Massachusetts General Hospital (MGH) shortly thereafter signed a $50 million, ten-year contract with the West German–French firm Hoechst-Roussel for molecular-biology research. MGH has academic freedom guarantees. In return Hoechst has an opportunity to capitalize on discoveries before others, and to obtain exclusive licenses to develop resultant products.[28]

Another side to the conflict-of-interest issue was presented in a recent *New England Journal of Medicine* editorial by Arnold Relman. Entrepreneurialism in medicine is rampant, he said. Research with potential commercial applications attracts corporate and venture capitalist interests. Therefore, reports in journals or at meetings may cause substantial fluctuations in stock prices, as has happened in more than one instance with articles published in the *Journal*. In wrestling with what the *Journal*'s stance should be, the editor and his assistants developed the policy that manuscripts should be selected solely on the basis of their merits and suitability for the *Journal*, and not with regard to authors' commercial associations or presumed motivation. Rather, the *Journal* will suggest to authors that they routinely acknowledge all funding sources and relevant direct business associations in a footnote. Relman conceded that associations that are less clear or direct, such as part-time consulting, stock or other equity ownership in a firm, or patent-licensing agreements are more complicated; therefore, footnoted acknowledgment will need to be decided on a case-by-case basis.[29]

By now, Harvard's patent policy changes are woven tightly into the university's fabric. Faculty acceptance was prompted by several factors. First, the economics of medical care were changing. Second, according to Davis, attitudes at federal granting agencies shifted toward encouraging universities to patent federally funded research. Culliton identifies a few more motives: a wish to receive dollars free of federal regulations, and to deflect increasing federal influence on research directions. Regulations were viewed as time-consuming and inconsistent. Capitation—federal funds provided to schools to increase medical school class size—were intended to stave off a perceived doctor shortage. But the shortage and the capitation funds disappeared almost as suddenly as they had appeared, leaving schools with swollen faculties, inflated tuitions, and a new problem for society—the doctor glut.

University officials complained of other instances of overregulation. Circular A-21 required federal grant recipients to account for all their time, separating out the purposely commingled activities of teaching, research, and service. Grants in certain politically high-priority research areas were funded over those considered equally meritorious from a scientific standpoint. Not discussed by Culliton but also viewed with alarm was the increasing use of contract mechanisms to fund research of special interest to the granting agencies.

Harvard's new patent policies are not unique. Rather, they reflect a widespread trend. University actions are further complicated by uncertain patent office determinations in the field of cell biology. For instance, as Reid Adler recently described in *Science,* patent specification claims (which essentially define the scope of protection afforded by the patent) carry only a rebuttable presumption of validity; therefore, their allowance by the Patent and Trademark Office may be challenged and effectively second-guessed through litigation. In addition to opposing doctrines of legal interpretation, Adler describes patent litigation as an inexact science. When infringement is detected, suits may be reduced to expert witness debates. According to Adler, uncertainties about the likely scope of patent coverage awarded will affect business decisions to file for a patent or to preserve secrecy until court rulings better define the situation.[30]

Universities and commercial firms alike are affected by these uncertainties. Stanford developed an aggressive stance seeking a broad patent for a scientific hybrid plasmid used to transfer genes from one cell to another. The gene-splicing technique was developed in microorganisms by Stanley Cohen of Stanford and Herbert Boyer of U.C. San Francisco. The Patent Office granted Stanford rights for the *process* of making proteins with the hybrid plasmid, which has generated about $2.7 million from licensing fees; but the Patent Office only recently granted Stanford rights to *products* developed from these techniques. Because the application is one of the first filed relating to gene-splicing techniques, it is considered a test case. Initially the Patent Office rejected the claim, questioning whether the information it contained allowed others to duplicate the same product, as is required. The rejection also was based on questions of whether a third scientist, a former collaborator with Cohen and Boyer, should have been named as a coinventor.[31] These questions now answered in Stanford's favor, Stanford and UCSF will share equally in the process and product patent revenues until 1997.

Columbia University, in contrast, easily got a patent for both a process and the products resulting from it. The process, called cotransformation, was developed by Richard Axel of Columbia. With this technique for synthesizing products in large quantities, two or more unrelated genes are moved simultaneously into mammalian cells *in vitro.*[32] It is expected to be a more efficient means for protein synthesis than current methods using bacteria. The biomedical community now wonders whether this ruling covering both process and product represents a more liberal patent trend.

Trade-Secret Status Complications

The Cohen-Boyer example brings into question another aspect of patent uncertainties—the effect that publishing in journals and reporting at meetings on the results of research will have on potentially patentable products. This was one of the concerns of Harvard faculty in turning down the idea of forming a Harvard company. The problem relates not only to patents but also to trade-secret status of data.

Trade secrets, as explained by Adler, encompass private proprietary data or materials providing a competitive advantage to their owner. He cites as trade-secret examples hybridization conditions, cell lines, merchandizing plans, or customer lists. Trade secrets differ from patents in that they are potentially unlimited in duration, are regulated in most instances by state law, and are not required to satisfy the more stringent requirements of patent law. Courts can order compensation for unauthorized use of trade secrets discovered by improper means, such as breach of confidence. But trade secrets cannot be protected when they become public knowledge through independent discovery or disclosure, as through published articles or discussion. Threatening trade-secret status of data, therefore, are many of the usual means of doing business (in this case, conducting research) at universities. This includes the traditional freedom of scientific communication, prodded by academic pressure to publish and by the frequent movement of graduate students to new faculty positions elsewhere once they have completed their training, and stimulated by the use of meetings and workshops to advance knowledge and share ideas and information.[33]

Trade-secret status of data can be, however unintentionally, a formidable barrier to progress. One such example concerns an orphan drug, as related by the drug's developer, Jess Thoene of the University of Michigan. He was studying cystinosis, an extremely rare but fatal disorder, which occurs in no more than 1 in 50,000 live births. Cystinosis, or the accumulation of the amino acid cystine in cells, including those of the kidney, causes death from kidney malfunction in children by the time they are about ten years old. The only available therapy has been kidney dialysis, but Thoene found that the chemical cysteamine seemed to stabilize this process and possibly to improve kidney function.

He and his colleague, Jerry Schneider from the University of California, San Diego, applied for an emergency IND for cysteamine to treat the critically advanced stage of cystinosis in a child whose religion would not permit dialysis. Treated with cysteamine, the child's cell cystine content was initially lowered. Later, however, the child suffered a convulsive seizure, and therapy was discontinued. FDA thereupon requested additional information on cysteamine safety. While attempting to gather information on the chemical's synthesis, purity, and other characteristics during the next two years, Thoene learned of a Master File on cysteamine at FDA, which had been submitted by the chemical's supplier. Thoene, though acknowledging the need for trade secrets on commercial grounds, was astounded to learn that FDA, because of the trade-secret status of the Master File, had not told him of its existence so he could contact the supplier directly for information. After this two-year delay, Thoene was able to satisfy safety requirements and was allowed by FDA to continue trials with the drug. An FDA screen, however, then found a potential cancer-causing property of cysteamine. Since the carcinogen was the starting material from which cysteamine was synthesized, FDA would not reveal the identity of the carcinogen to Thoene.

FDA's reason was that disclosure would violate the trade secret of cysteamine manufacture. Thoene, who had learned from other sources about the Master File, called the president of the company involved and described his predicament. The president volunteered the necessary information on cysteamine synthesis. Thereafter, Thoene was able to demonstrate that the carcinogen is part of a water-soluble compound, which breaks down in water. Since the drug is taken in a water suspension, he began studies to determine whether this form of the drug had an acceptably low carcinogen level, which is set at less than 10 parts per million. Learning of Thoene's problems, the GPIA (Generic Pharmaceutical Industry Association) volunteered to underwrite the remaining costs of the cysteamine study.[34] In this case, breach of trade secrets was done voluntarily by their owner to aid an orphan-drug effort. The extent to which trade secrets will be revealed for orphan drug purposes remains uncertain, however, and FDA appears to be legally unable to help. The trade-off of the need to protect versus the need to know is particularly difficult in cases such as this one, where the proprietary information is intended to be used for an unprofitable product. It seems, however, that FDA officials aware of such situations could intervene directly with sponsors to determine whether the sponsor would be willing to cooperate with the orphan-drug developer.

Despite risks of trade-secret information leaks, reliance on trade secrets rather than patents may be prudent, since, according to Adler, the rapid pace of research may render patents outdated even before they are issued.

His advice is exemplified, to some extent, by the case of insulin. Eli Lilly's standard insulin brand has dominated the market since its introduction in the 1920s. Recently, however, the product was challenged by a purified pork insulin made by two Danish firms. Lilly countered by manufacturing its own purified form and concurrently initiated attempts to produce human insulin in bacteria with the biotechnology firm Genentech. If they are successful, the new product may offer advantages over purified animal-derived insulin. The human form might be easier to produce; it might be less expensive; it would not be subject to animal supply problems; and it might be especially advantageous for those numerous patients who respond poorly to bovine or porcine insulin.

The diabetes field itself may be changing, however. Subcutaneous pumps for insulin administration are being used to infuse insulin in amounts calibrated to the body's exact needs; since "clumping" is a problem, these may require insulin prepared to the pump's specific requirements. Researchers, exploring still another approach, are experimenting with transplanting entire pancreases between animals, or just transplanting the islets of Langerhans (the body's insulin-producing cells) isolated from the pancreas. Scientists are trying to determine whether tissue rejection problems can be overcome acceptably, especially with drugs such as cyclosporin. Scientists are also trying to determine whether transplantation will result in natural insulin regulation. Finally, they will be assessing whether transplantation halts capillary basement-membrane thickening, which occurs early in the course of the disease and may be responsible for or related to major vascular complications, including premature atherosclerosis, retinopathy, neuropathy, and gangrene. Successful answers in animals might lead to human transplantation.[35] Although pancreas or islet cell transplantation might not become the treatment of choice, the example illustrates the rapidly accelerating technological pace in which drug developers are making decisions on products that may be a decade away from marketability. During that period the field might change so radically that these products may be rendered obsolete before they are marketed. New technologies and responses to them by industry and academia all have substantive consequences for orphan drugs.

Some Implications for Orphan Drugs

Stochastic opinion and conjecture suggest that molecular-biology technologies may affect development of orphan drugs in several interconnected ways, both technologically and commercially. Scientists using recombinant DNA and monoclonal antibody techniques may be able to identify and synthesize therapeutic agents to counteract disease-producing molecular abnormalities. This could be a lot cheaper and more effective than the previous practice of screening thousands of chemicals for possible biological activity and testing them for therapeutic properties. Additionally, molecular biology may aid both in determining defects that are responsible for diseases and disorders, and in designing synthetic agents to ameliorate or replace defective "parts." The process could result in less toxic therapies, which are more effective, less time-consuming to develop, more likely to win FDA approval, and therefore perhaps more commercially attractive despite small markets. Third, patent rulings concerning recombinant DNA and monoclonal antibody techniques may confer new forms of market protection, perhaps circumventing current problems with unpatentable natural substances. In fact, unpatentable drugs generally may get market relief from current patent-term legislation (to be discussed in later chapters).

The following examples depict an optimistic orphan-drug scenario. Stanley Prusiner at the University of California, San Francisco, and his colleagues recently reported isolating a defective gene in an animal model of multiple sclerosis, a neurological disorder affecting about 200,000 people in the United States. Its characteristic is breakdown of myelin (insulation) surrounding nerve fibers (the wiring) in the brain, which is expressed as episodes of symptoms and subsequent remissions. The finding of this abnormality represented one of the first direct links between a specific genetic defect and a neurological disorder in mammals. Although the work is still in early stages, these scientists hypothesize that multiple sclerosis represents an immune reaction to the abnormal myelin protein produced by the defective gene. This would open the way for detection of the presence of the defective gene in utero, as now can be done with certain lipid-storage diseases using amniocentesis (drawing amniotic fluid samples from the sack enveloping the fetus). Scientists also speculate that eventually the disease might be prevented by replacing or correcting the defective gene.[36]

A second example is the synthetic vaccine described earlier, which has been the subject of a bizarre patent struggle. Synthetic vaccines might have major safety advantages over killed-virus or live-attenuated-virus vaccines now in use. The purer, safer vaccines might steer a new course around the liability risks that currently threaten vaccine manufacturers.[37]

On the negative side, the scramble to develop commercially attractive products may redirect the attention of university researchers toward potential market winners. Development of orphan drugs, especially those that are expensive to produce, are unpatentable, or are intended for small markets, would be as much an opportunity cost to universities as to industry: In either case, funds would have to be diverted away from developing potential market "winners." Although some would claim that universities will always encourage pursuit of basic knowledge and of scientific answers to orphan as well as common diseases, the environment is too new for us to assess the merits of the consequences of these concerns. Nonetheless, as universities begin to depend more on industry sources of support, it seems appropriate to design a set of attractive market and regulatory incentives for both industry and academia, or, at least, incentives that make the situation less unattractive.

Notes

1. National Science Foundation, *University-Industry Research Relationships*, NDB 82-1 (Washington, D.C.: U.S. Government Printing Office, 1982), pp. 11–28.

2. Ibid., pp. 2–7, 27.

3. David Schwartzman, *Innovation in the Pharmaceutical Industry* (Baltimore, Md.: Johns Hopkins University Press, 1976), pp. 54–57.

4. Fred Karch, ed., *Orphan Drugs* (New York: Marcel Dekker, 1982), pp. 1–205.

5. Leon Goldberg and John Zaroslinski, "Development of Dopamine," in Karch, *Orphan Drugs*, pp. 118–137.

6. Confidential personal communication.

7. Donald Griffith, presentation before the PMA Commission on Drugs for Rare Diseases, December 16, 1981.

8. J. M. Walshe, "Triethylene Tetramine Dihydrochloride," in Karch, *Orphan Drugs*, pp. 58–71.

9. Berton Roueché, "Annals of Medicine: Live and Let Live," *New Yorker*, July 16, 1979.

10. Melvin Van Woert, "L-5-Hydroxytryptophan," in Karch, *Orphan Drugs*, pp. 14–31.

11. *Evaluating and Patenting Faculty Inventions* (Tucson, Ariz.: Research Corporation), pp. 10–12; *Report for 1982* (Tucson, Ariz.: Research Corporation), p. 12.

12. Stephen De Felice, "The Carnitine Story," in Karch, *Orphan Drugs*, pp. 34–55.

13. James Stubbins, "Alkylating Local Anesthetics," in Karch, *Orphan Drugs*, pp. 74–87.

14. Majorie Sun, "NIH Ponders Pitfalls of Industrial Support," *Science* 213(1981):113–114.

15. National Science Foundation, "University-Industry Research Relationships," p. 15.

16. Leroy Randall, NIH Patent Office, personal communication, March 1984.

17. Marjorie Sun, "Dole Promotes Patent Reform for Big Business," *Science* 223(4633)(1984):264.

18. Sun, "Pitfalls," pp. 113–114.

19. Nicholas Wade, "La Jolla Biologists Troubled by the Midas Factor," *Science* 213(7)(1981):623–628.

20. B. J. Culliton, "Biomedical Research Enters the Marketplace," *New England Journal of Medicine*, May 14, 1981, pp. 1195–1201.

21. National Science Fondation, "University-Industry Research Relationships," pp. 15–16.

22. Government Accounting Office, *Assuring Reasonableness of Rising Indirect Costs on NIH Research Grants—A Difficult Problem* (Washington, D.C.: GAO/HRD 84-3, 1984).

23. Jeffrey L. Fox, "GAO Report Documents Rising Indirect Costs," *Science* 224(1984):267–268; Barbara Culliton, "NIH Seeks Reduction in 'Indirect Costs,'" *Science* 221(1983):929–930.

24. Ibid.

25. Lawrence Altman, "Physician's Move to Industry May Reflect Widening Trend," *New York Times*, July 28, 1981.

26. Culliton, "Biomedical Research," p. 1200.

27. Bernard Davis, "Sounding Board: Profit Sharing Between Professors and the University," *New England Journal of Medicine* 304(20)(1981):1232–1235.

28. Altman, "Physician's Move," *New York Times*.

29. Arnold Relman, "Dealing with Conflicts of Interest," *New England Journal of Medicine* 310(18)(1984):1182–1183.

30. Reid Adler, "Biotechnology as an Intellectual Property," *Science* 224(1984):357–363.

31. Marjorie Sun, "Cohen-Boyer Patent to Be Issued Soon," *Science* 224(4646)(1984):264.

32. Fox, "GAO Report."

33. Adler, "Biotechnology," p. 361.

34. Blanchard Hiatt, "Orphan Drugs, Orphan Diseases," *Research News* (University of Michigan) 33(8)(1982):4–6.

35. Marjorie Sun, "Insulin Wars: New Advances May Throw Market into Turbulence," *Science* 21(1980):1225—1228.

36. "Isolation of Nervous System Gene May Help Multiple Sclerosis Study," *Philadephia Inquirer*, May 1984.

37. Wade, "Midas Factor."

5
Efforts to Investigate and Efforts to Legislate Orphan Drugs

The 1970s and early 1980s were a time of several independent planning efforts by both public- and private-sector officials. Two federal interagency task forces were convened within a four-year interval to define the orphan-drug situation and propose solutions; several bills were introduced in Congress proposing federal initiatives; and the PMA reported it was working on industry plans for coming to grips with the problem.

Federal planning began as FDA sought measures to aid academic and federal orphan-drug developers in their previously disappointing quest for commercial drug sponsorship. Voluntary health agencies joined with researchers to lobby for solutions. The PMA reacted by announcing it was studying the problem but then retained a conspicuous public silence. Representative Elizabeth Holtzman (D-N.Y.), in response to urging by scientists and voluntary health agency members, introduced the first legislation specifically on orphan drugs in 1980. Moving testimony presented during hearings on the Holtzman bill by a young Los Angeles man named Adam Seligman, who suffers from Tourette syndrome, and a young New York wife and mother, Sharon Dobkin, who suffers from myoclonus, was to have far-reaching effects. Their comments, picked up by the *L.A. Times*, demonstrated the deep frustration of patients who see their hopes for therapeutic rescue held hostage to market demands.

The *L.A. Times'* article was brought to the attention of television's "Quincy," Jack Klugman, by his brother, Maurice. Within a year, the plight of orphan drugs, presented in a balanced yet dramatic show, was catapulted from an insider's dialogue conducted mainly in medical journals and federal offices to a nationally recognized tragedy. Orphan drugs suddenly had become what Donald Schön of MIT would call "an idea in good currency."[1]

As Schön describes them, ideas in good currency are those that are powerful enough to stimulate public policy. Such ideas start at the periphery and often, by the time they arrive in the mainstream, no longer accurately reflect the existing state of affairs. In reflecting on this paradox, Schön concludes that a principal criterion for effective learning is the social system's ability to reduce this lag time so that ideas in good currency do reflect current problems. Representatives Henry Waxman (D-Calif.) and Theodore Weiss (D-N.Y.) did precisely that. Waxman, chairman of the Subcommittee on Health and the Environment of the House Committee on Energy and Commerce, convened a hearing on Weiss's bill, a reintroduction of the Holtzman bill of the previous Congress. (Representative Holtzman had given up her House seat to run, unsuccessfully, for the Senate.) The hearing was held within days of the "Quincy" orphan-drug episode. This time, Adam Seligman was accompanied by the show's star, Jack Klugman. The actor reenacted from the witness table his congressional appearance scene from the show to argue on behalf of legislation for orphan drugs. In a brilliant instance of life imitating art, Klugman took industry and government to task in full public view before a crowded press section and television cameras. Federal and industry orphan-drug efforts immediately began to speed up. Before this dramatic stimulant to public awareness of orphan drug problems, however, much had transpired to lay a foundation for action.

The 1974 Federal Interagency Task Force

The U.S. government, which back in 1964 had laid to rest concerns that PHS hospitals might not receive adequate supplies of drugs through industry public-service products, decided to reexplore the situation of drugs with limited commercial value. In 1969 the PMA had updated its list of service drugs, which included a total of thirty-nine products from fourteen PMA member companies. Most drugs were available as Compassionate INDs. T. Donald Rucker, Social Security Administration official (now at Ohio State University), had proposed a joint government-industry study of the problem in 1970, but one was never undertaken, according to a report by Kemp.[2]

Three years later interest expressed during an HEW Executive Committee meeting reopened the investigation. Subsequent inquiries turned up the existence of the 1964 committee report and the PMA drug lists. This material was used as background for the newly formed DHEW Interagency Task Force, convened by FDA and chaired by Marion Finkel, then associate director for new drug evaluation, Bureau of Drugs.

Task force participants primarily were administrators of federal orphan-drug programs such as those in CDC, NCI, and NINCDS. They formed six study groups. Study Group I was to define the limited-use drug problem, its scope and importance to public health. The other groups saw their tasks as dependent on those of Group I; ultimately, this led to a premature end to the planning.

Group II was to determine the feasibility of various economic incentives for pharmaceutical companies to carry out the development and distribution of orphan drugs. Group III was to weigh pros and cons of a government service to develop orphan drugs; Group IV was to consider the legalities of industry use of government patents and the provision of federally funded data to industry in support of a patent. Group V was to explore the feasibility of obtaining liability insurance for clinical testing, and Group VI was charged with examining problems attending drugs owned or originated by foreign firms.

Although all the groups were to work simultaneously, Groups II through VI awaited the outcome of Group I's problem definition. As Kemp noted in his report from Group I to the task force, the lack of an information base substantially undermined attempts to understand the issues and develop policies. Kemp reported that Group I found allusions to individual problems but could locate no systematic information or analysis of the nature and extent of the problem. Thus Group I's efforts ground to a halt, with the other groups backed up right behind it.

The task force's interim report advanced these conclusions: (1) that data were inadequate to determine the number and type of patients who might benefit from access to orphan drugs; and (2) that without this information, the task force was reluctant to suggest meaningful policy recommendations. Still, the report contained some general recommendations of study groups:

1. The solution of choice would range from the optimal—no government intervention—to the least acceptable—continuous government intervention.
2. It is the obligation of society, as represented by government, to make important medical drugs available to those who need them.
3. Additional efforts should be made to study the problem.

Moreover, the task force did make planning recommendations:

1. The task force should compile a list of drugs fitting the "limited commercial value" profile.
2. The list should be published in the Federal Register to alert

manufacturers about the wish of FDA to work with prospective sponsors.

3. The task force report should be transmitted to higher levels of management to seek endorsement and gain guidance and encouragement for continued FDA activity.[3]

According to FDA officials, however, because there had been no definition of the problem, the report was never advanced through channels, and no formal action was taken on these three recommendations.

The 1978 Interagency Task Force

A second Interagency Task Force was convened following inquiries by some members of Congress and by Peter Bourne, former special advisor to President Carter on health affairs, according to Marion Finkel of the FDA.[4]

Their interest was sparked by recommendations made by the congressionally mandated Commission on the Control of Huntingtons Disease and its Consequences.[5] The commission was chaired by Marjorie Guthrie, who, depending on the generation of the people she was addressing, would introduce herself either as folk singer Woody Guthrie's widow or as Arlo Guthrie's mother. Woody had died of the disease; Arlo, like every other child born to a Huntington disease victim, has a 50 percent chance of inheriting it. Huntingtons disease was a paradigm for exploring the range of problems common to rare diseases: It is rare. It is genetically determined, but onset of symptoms does not begin until the fourth decade or later. The disease, which causes severe physical and mental deterioration, has no effective therapy, no effective means of in utero diagnosis, and no symptomatic treatment. Guthrie and Nancy Wexler, the commission's executive director, used Huntingtons as a model to focus the commission's recommendations on the broad problems besetting rare diseases in general. The commission came out strongly in favor of increased efforts in basic neurological research applicable to rare diseases, including drug R&D, and emphasized this message during congressional hearings on the commission's findings.

Pressure to convene a second Task Force also came from FDA's Neurologic Drugs Advisory Committee, which had heard of the difficulties faced by Melvin Van Woert, John Walshe, and others and had recommended a coordinated agency approach, according to Marion Finkel's opening remarks to the 1978 task force members. She reviewed comments of the earlier task force, explained the problem of lack of data they faced, and encouraged the current members—again, primarily federal and university scientists and a PMA liaison—to propose recommendations, even if it was difficult to provide an exact definition of what constituted drugs of limited commercial value.[6]

Reportedly FDA officials had requested industry participation, but invitations were declined. In the meantime, according to PMA's John Adams, an industry group was meeting independently to explore the issues and to develop a new list of service drugs.[7]

In the absence of pharmaceutical-industry participation, the task force sought to anticipate the financial incentives desired and to propose administrative and legislative means for providing them. The task force format, according to some participants, consisted of a single overview session during which individual federal administrators discussed difficulties with orphan drugs known to their agencies. This was followed by a meeting of some subgroups. Thereafter, a report was written under contract by a consultant-lawyer from the Research Institute of the American Arbitration Association. The report, released in 1979, was summarized by Marion Finkel.[8]

The essence of the program proposed by the 1978 task force was a voluntary effort to stimulate development of certain orphan drugs, specifically those deemed by an advisory board to be valuable therapeutically but not financially. The report focused on drugs for rare diseases but included comments regarding unpatentable drugs and those with high liability risks.

The proposed program would be based on economic, scientific, and legal incentives to industry. Profits realized from those incentives, however, would be returned in whole or in part to government. Thus the federal role would be that of a facilitator or broker, using broad negotiating powers rather than providing direct subsidy. Specific policy and procedure would be decided on a case-by-case basis by the independent advisory board, which was to be located, initially at least, within the FDA. The board would serve as advisor, through the FDA commissioner, to the DHHS secretary.[9]

Incentives would fall within three categories: (1) administrative and organizational, (2) financial and commercial, and (3) "recognitional." As an administrative incentive, FDA would give priority to orphan drugs in the review process. As organizational incentives, according to the report, arrangements that do not conflict with antitrust laws or noncompetitive activity contrary to the public interest would be encouraged. These included voluntary consortia to share risk, facility, or liability costs; contracts between commercial and nonprofit organizations for drug sponsorship; partnerships; and exchange of rights of ownership patents, licenses, or other assets.

Financial and commercial incentives included suggestions for government purchase of orphan drugs, and various loans to developers (low interest, variable interest, long-term, variable term, minimal security, cost-sharing, or stipulated forgiveness). According to the report, this would require legislation to establish a revolving fund with periodic infusion of public and private dollars. Additionally, the report suggested use of grants and contracts for orphan-drug R&D with the stipulation that contracts would include cost-sharing or joint-venture agreements and automatic payback for drugs that proved to be profitable.

Suggested legislative incentives included: authorization for the loans just described; tax advantages (allowances, depreciation, deductions) for costs and expenses; amendment of patent laws to allow exclusive or modified patents or licenses; amendment of antitrust laws to permit limited exchange of data, pooling, and other collaboration; and amendments to FDA law to provide grants and contract authority where these were not then available. The report emphasized that this voluntary method would succeed only with the dedicated cooperation of all concerned parties.

The task force brought to the public the first systematic plan for addressing the orphan-drug situation. Many of the ideas, especially legislative proposals such as tax incentives and patent protection provisions, appeared promising. Some provisions were troubling, however. One contradiction seemed to be the requirement for repaying incentive or subsidy costs if drugs should become profitable through expanded uses or other means. The most compelling market incentive for developing orphan drugs is the possibility that the drug might be found useful in other indications and thus increase market value. A payback ruling might discourage sponsors from seeking a supplemental NDA for these new uses and risking a payback requirement since the drug already would be on the market and available for any use. Moreover, with the payback provision, the incentive hardly would seem equal to the opportunity costs incurred by diverting time and money away from other products in favor of the orphan project.

Administrative provisions seemed sound but hardly new. Benefit/risk assessment is a factor in all drug approval decisions, not a new thrust to be applied to orphan drugs. Why not have early pre-

IND talks with sponsors of all new drugs, not just sponsors of orphan drugs? Time spent by FDA reviewers at this stage might decrease the time needed later for drug application reviews. This question was raised in subsequent debate.[10] Also questioned were legislative suggestions concerning tax advantages or alternatives to existing patent constraints. These, though appealing, had been proposed without evaluation of feasibility or consequences—especially those involving antitrust changes—by congressional staff of subcommittees dealing with these areas of authority. Therefore, viability of many of the task force recommendations seemed dubious. An additional question was how to deal with the possible conflict of interest that might arise if the nation's regulatory agency were to become a drug developer through new authority to provide grants or contracts, or were to house and staff an independent advisory board.

The major concern was the planning format and some of the underlying assumptions on the basis of which incentives were proposed. It is difficult for federal representatives to try to devise plans for industry participation with industry absent from the deliberations. Studies in using the systems approach suggest that "stakeholder" planning—that is, participation by those affecting or affected by the system at issue—carries several advantages.[11]

First, the range of stakeholders often represent diverse points of view and expertise. This allows a more informed and comprehensive evaluation of proposals. Second, those who participate in creating policy are more apt to make it work. Third, broader participation can provide a look at the larger system of which orphan drugs are a part. Changes that may seem infeasible when one looks only at orphan drugs may become viable alternatives in the context of changes in the system as a whole. Finally, problems attending orphan drugs may have a greater chance for resolution (reaching a compromise, with both sides winning some points and losing others) or dissolution (making changes in the larger system so that the problem no longer exists) if both industry and government are party to the planning, as described by Russell Ackoff and Fred Emery of the Wharton School, two of the developers of the systems approach.[12] Among supporters of stakeholder participation in the health field are economists Roger Battistella of Cornell and Steven Eastaugh of George Washington University, who suggest that key interest groups that are a party to decisions in the reorganized British national health service are more apt to accept and implement them.[13]

These are simply alternative proposals for the process of policymaking; the Interagency Task Force chose a different one. However, several additional concerns remain. First, the Task Force report acknowledged the preceding group's call for additional data; according to the report, however, action—not more study—was needed now. Although unquestionably action was needed, so, it seemed, was further study. If lack of incentives was deemed the primary obstruction for orphan drugs, then policy might stand better informed by investigating whether incentives would have the same or different effects on small and large firms, especially with regard to differences in fixed versus variable costs and in means of liability coverage. Additionally, could any inferences be drawn on needed incentives by comparing successful orphan candidates with unsuccessful ones to date?

Finally, the fact that industry had been invited to participate and had declined had definite policy implications. The planning in isolation that occurred with the federal task force and the corresponding PMA discussion are characteristic of parties in conflict. As Ackoff and Emery describe, if B's presence *decreases* the expected value of A's state, then the parties are in conflict; if B's presence *increases* the expected value of A's state, they are in cooperation.[14] Comments on orphan drugs from industry and government alike had suggested that the groups agreed on common ends—that is, that technically feasible medical drugs should be developed and made available to people who need them—suggesting the environment was ripe for cooperative policymaking. Yet from the planning posture exhibited by industry, it appeared that PMA member companies expected to be in conflict with government over designing means to those ends. The task force, in ignoring this adversarial stance, devised incentives predicated on cooperation without proposing means for creating a more cooperative environment. There was very little attention to devising means for improving coordination between activities of the FDA and those of federal research agencies, or better communication between these agencies and industry. Finally, the task force suggestions appeared characteristic of arbitration situations, wherein both groups agree to have a third party hear and determine the case in controversy. But unless industry viewed the incentives as worthwhile enough to induce them to bring cases before the proposed advisory board, there might be a few cases to arbitrate.

In fact, neither the assumption that cooperation would obtain nor that industry desired market incentives was based on clear-cut indications from industry. Company officials' comments regarding the first assumption suggested the existence of an adversarial rather than a cooperative atmosphere. Comments on incentives were mixed.

For instance, a 1980 GAO report seeking to define reasons for the slowness of the drug approval process credited its apparent glacial pace to the adversarial relationship between FDA and industry, as well as to factors such as intense congressional and consumer scrutiny and a conservative regulatory approach. GAO staff reported that FDA officials were viewed by those in industry as favoring this adversarial stance.[15] Pfizer's president, Gerald Laubach, wrote that although antagonism is not legislated into the FDA role, the one-sidedness of the agency's mandate encourages skepticism toward drugs and their manufacturers.[16] Arthur Levin of New York University stressed the need for consensus rather than the current adversarial environment in the health field in general. Thomas Althius, a Pfizer vice-president, published a list of forty drugs with annual sales of less than $3 million as evidence of the industry's socially responsible actions; and suggested that a cooperative rather than an adversarial relationship between government, academia, and industry would be a constructive first step toward more rational drug regulation, benefiting all drugs, including those considered to be orphans.[17]

During semistructured, open-ended interviews conducted by the author with top officials of FDA and of seven major pharmaceutical firms, there was unanimity in characterizing the FDA-industry relationship as adversarial.[18] A few FDA and industry officials qualified their statements by saying the stance is exaggerated at times to demonstrate the absence of collusion. Industry officials attributed FDA's adversary position to several factors. First was the nature of agency members, some of whom were thought to be reactionary and overzealous in carrying out the mission of protection but not in expediting approval of important new therapies. A second factor was congressional oversight pressure. Third was bureaucratic inefficiency, including serial rather than simultaneous review of the various sections in IND and NDA applications, and frequent personnel turnovers, which produced long delays and inconsistencies between recommendations of prior and present reviewers. Fourth was an active pursuit by FDA of policies considered by some industry officials to overextend the agency's role in fostering competition. A few officials contended that the adversarial relationship was productive: It often resulted in better applications, based on FDA reviewer's comments; and it forced difficult but necessary benefit/risk judgments to be made.

Comments from FDA officials and drug reviewers suggested industry actions sometimes promote an adversarial response. Industry was cited as often submitting incomplete applications, with the intention of initiating the review process prematurely before in-house drug assessment had been completed. Others suggested that industry sponsors use FDA reviewers inappropriately, seeking advice on whether the company should continue to pursue a drug candidate based on the data obtained and presented to FDA. Still others felt industry invested too much effort in trying to speed up FDA review—effort that might have been invested in better presentation of data to enable reviewers to assess their merits more easily.

Specifically regarding orphan drugs, industry officials differed among themselves on some issues and agreed on others. For instance, many officials considered the major orphan problems to apply to drugs for women and children, because of high liability risks, and to involve diseases for which no effective drugs have been found because no leads exist. Some industry officials did not consider small market by itself to be a disincentive, especially if patent protection were available, if liability risks were not considered greater than average, and if means for determining efficacy were well worked out. Others felt that small market was disincentive enough, especially for large firms with high fixed costs.

Finally, views were mixed on whether the industry should provide orphan drugs solely as a function of social responsibility. Some supported the economic position of Milton Friedman, advising that industry is strong by virtue of the profits it amasses and can return to R&D to support national development. Specifically, Friedman argued corporate social responsibility should be avoided insofar as such actions reduce returns to stockholders, raise prices to consumers, or lower employee wages. To do otherwise is to spend money that does not belong to the corporation.[19] Executives who hold the Friedman view strongly favored tax benefits for orphan-drug development, and some form of market exclusivity for unpatentable drugs. Other officials seemed to view the issue more in the terms expressed by Battistella and Eastaugh.[20] They wrote that trying to achieve social responsibility in health services using marketplace principles, derived from highly reductionistic economic models, can lead to a wrong diagnosis and a treatment that is worse than the disease. These officials said the industry will continue to develop and distribute orphan drugs as a social responsibility, as it has in the past, because society has provided industry with profit margins and industry should be willing to return some of these benefits to society. They emphasized the need for streamlined FDA processes to expedite review of all drugs, both orphan and nonorphan, and the need for improved channels of communication and working relationships with academia on orphan-drug projects. They said, in essence, that they should not have to pay unnecessarily for the privilege of holding this viewpoint.

S. 1075: The National Office for Drug Science

At approximately the same time as the 1978 task force deliberations, the Senate Health and Scientific Research Subcommittee of the Committee on Labor and Human Resources was considering drug regulation reform. Senator Edward Kennedy (D-Mass.) and six co-sponsors introduced S.1075, an amendment to the Public Health Act, to revise and reform federal law applicable to drugs for human and other use. According to Senator Kennedy's statement on the Senate floor in introducing the bill, one major motive was the need for research and development on drugs for developing nations.[21]

Under Title II of the bill, a National Office for Drug Science was to be established. Originally termed "Center," it was renamed "Office" because the former sounded too bureaucratic, according to a staff aide to former Senator Jacob Javits (R-N.Y.).[22] The proposed office was to contain a division of policy and research as well as one for clinical-pharmacology and clinical-pharmacy training. The divisions would be able to conduct and support research, either by request or on their own initiative into the safety and effectiveness of FDA-approved drugs; the development of drugs for diseases and other conditions of low incidence; and potential drug science research breakthroughs. Section 1082 provided for the office to publish its intentions concerning specific drugs in the Federal Register prior to initiating projects. (The PMA intended to challenge the need for any drug development effort that was announced, according to PMA vice-president John Adams.)[23]

The office was to have a program of drug science policy research to review and analyze three areas: (1) the impact of regulation on drug innovation and development; (2) problems posed by risk/benefit analyses, formulation of such ratios, and their use in approving drugs; and (3) methods for improving and accelerating drug research, innovation, development, investigation, approval, and utilization processes. The initial appropriation proposed was $5 million for the fiscal year ending September 30, 1981, and would increase by $2 million for each of the next two years, ending at $9 million for the fiscal year ending September 30, 1983.[24]

According to a Kennedy staff member, there was little discussion by concerned parties of the Office for Drug Science proposed in the bill, although other provisions for regulatory reform contained in the bill generated considerable lobbying efforts. Apparently the only unofficial comments about the office from FDA officials concerned their aversion to its possible "policing" image. NIH officials unofficially feared the office might result in diversion of federal funds from basic research into drug R&D. There was no input during the bill's drafting or markup stages by members of the Interagency Task Force.[25] The bill passed the Senate but was not acted on by the House.

H.R. 7089: The First Orphan-Drug Legislation

Although the 1978 task force report had not considered how the underlying (but not explicit) assumptions might affect the success of the task force plan, the approach was innovative and systematic. Since industry had not come forth with a plan of its own, it was the only publicly available blueprint.

When Melvin Van Woert and members of the National Myoclonus Foundation eventually appealed to Representative Holtzman for help, they explained that neither industry nor the NIH nor the FDA had been able to devise a means for making L-5HPT affordable for clinical trials, for securing an NDA, or for making the drug commercially available. After learning from industry and government representatives that the allegations of Van Woert were correct, Representative Holtzman decided to seek a legislative solution and turned to the interagency report for guidance on the kind of bill to draft.

H.R. 7089 was introduced on April 17, 1980. It provided for an Office of Drugs of Limited Commercial Value to be established at NIH to assist in the development of drugs for diseases or conditions of low incidence. Representative Holtzman had decided to move the proposed Office from FDA to the NIH to avoid any potential problems of conflict of interest. J. Richard Crout, director of the FDA Bureau of Drugs (now in charge of NIH's Research Applications office) already had commented on the advisability of giving NIH the lead in dealing with problems of orphan drugs.[26]

The office, as outlined in the Holtzman bill, would have a nine-member advisory council appointed by the NIH director, including members of the pharmaceutical industry, medical profession, scientific community, and public interest groups. The council was to propose recommendations to shorten drug approval time. It also would have the authority to provide financial assistance or other help in developing certain drugs, to purchase liability insurance for developers, to coordinate public and private efforts, and to collect information. Financial recipients were to reimburse the government for all or part of the expended funds if the drug's revenue exceeded the levels specified when funds first were made available. Drugs for diseases of low incidence to be covered under the act were those with limited commercial value that were unavailable because estimated sales revenues were judged insufficient for drug development without federal assistance, estimated sales revenues were judged insufficient to establish safety and efficacy, or exclusive development rights could not be obtained.[27]

At the hearing on the Holtzman bill on June 16, 1980, Representative Henry Waxman, chairman of the House Subcommittee on Health and the Environment, characterized the orphan-drug problem as a priority issue of the subcommittee. No industry officials testified at the hearing. Testimony was presented by FDA officials, scientists, voluntary agency officials, and some patients with rare diseases, including Tourette syndrome patient Adam Seligman. Like Huntingtons disease, Tourette syndrome is rare, it has a genetic susceptibility, and it is classified as a neuropsychiatric disorder.[28] Tourette syndrome produces involuntary movements, grunts, and vocalizations that frequently are obscene. As Seligman related, it can be debilitating; and, as he demonstrated, it takes enormous courage to persevere in public. Haloperidol, marketed by McNeil Pharmaceutical (of Johnson & Johnson) has been the drug of choice for treating Tourette syndrome, but its effectiveness varies from patient to patient and its side effects can be severe. Pimozide has been used for Tourette syndrome in Europe and Canada, but had not been approved for use in the United States. Seligman, who had not responded well to Haloperidol, had been smuggling in pimozide for his own use. On one occasion his supply of the drug was confiscated at customs, as is usual with all nonapproved drugs found being brought into the country. McNeil had been studying pimozide for possible use in schizophrenia and extended the trials to Tourette syndrome. The company, however, had discontinued the schizophrenia trials and reportedly planned to drop those on Tourette syndrome too.

The Holtzman bill had not elicited much enthusiasm from government or industry officials. The absence of authorization in the bill for specific appropriations earmarked for the proposed NIH office's functions, as well as perceived difficulties in devising means to carry out the specified activities, served to diminish NIH officials' interest. According to the PMA's John Adams, industry maintained its opposition to greater entry by government in the drug business, preferring to retain the option to address orphan-drug problems—if they did exist—themselves.

Although no action was taken on the Holtzman bill that year (1980) several other bills were introduced. A few of those that passed during the 96th Congress (1979-1981) were considered to have potential for affecting orphan drugs. Enacted legislation included the

1980 Stevenson-Wydler Technology Innovation Act (P.L. 96-480) to provide support for innovation and technology transfer, including funds for industry-university cooperative research projects. P.L. 96-517, the Uniform Federal Patent Policy Act of 1980, amended the patent and trademark laws to allow for transfer or assignment of rights for federally funded inventions to universities or small businesses involved in their development, as described in the previous chapter. A related measure, enacted in the 97th Congress, was the Small Business Innovation Act of 1982 (P.L. 97-219), designed to stimulate small and minority business involvement in federally funded research and development, and to encourage commercialization of federally funded R&D innovations. NIH's budget under the act is the second largest among the eleven federal agencies covered. During the law's authorized six-year life span, NIH funding will increase from 0.2 percent of its extramural (grants and contracts) budget to 1.5 percent for the sixth year. First-year funds in FY 1983 totaled $6.55 million, whereas FY 1984 funds, in keeping with the escalating scale, equal $20.7 million. However, the implications of this act for orphan drugs are not clear. As yet, no applications for orphan-drug projects have successfully competed for funding.[29]

In his powerful appearance before the Waxman subcommittee hearings on the Weiss bill in 1981, television actor Jack Klugman emphasized that although there were no villains in the orphan-drug dilemma, there were also no heroes—only innocent victims. These included, he said, people like Adam Seligman and Sharon Dobkin, whose testimony on the Holtzman bill in the previous Congress had inspired the "Quincy" episode. Their collective tragedy, he added, was embodied in the TV drama's victim, portrayed as a young man with Tourette syndrome who died running away from the public humiliation of his disease. Klugman asked where the dividing line was between those who get help and those who do not. Everybody, he said, had to carry some of the burden.

Seligman then summed up the situation. Basically, he said, the issue of orphan drugs has not been dealth with. He described going to Canada and Europe to get pimozide, including one instance when it was confiscated at customs. Initially, he said, he got good results with the drug, but later side effects caused him to stop using it. Now he was not using anything. His tics will get worse, he said; soon he will be grunting obscenities and twisting and twitching, and there will be very little he can do about it.[30] The two men's messages were simple and strong. Klugman's appearance was featured on that night's evening news and in the next day's newspapers.

A *Wall Street Journal* editorial, "Leave of Reality," likened Klugman's appearance before the subcommittee as an orphan-drug expert to that of asking Leonard Nimoy ("Star Trek's" Mr. Spock) to testify on the space program or Mary Tyler Moore, (who portrayed a television news production assistant to "Mr. Grant") to discuss discrimination against women in the workplace. The *Journal's* bottom line was that actors should not be set up as authorities on real-life issues such as public policy and commerce.[31] Nevertheless, Klugman's appearance, coming right on the heels of the "Quincy" dramatization, was probably the single most important catalyst in the entire orphan-drug saga.

Pimozide, the drug Seligman mentioned, exemplified many of the elements of the orphan-drug problem, as described in testimony of David Collins, then president of McNeil. The company, which has been investigating several orphan-drug uses, had secured market approval for haloperidol (Haldol) for use in schizophrenia and Tourette syndrome in 1967. The company initiated studies on pimozide in schizophrenia in the late 1960s. By 1977 pimozide was marketed abroad and was used by physicians in foreign countries with apparent success in patients with Tourette syndrome, according to Collins. Clinical investigators in this country wanted to initiate clincial trials for this indication; four studies undertaken from 1977 through 1979 were still in progress at the time of the hearings. McNeil did not sponsor its own investigation of pimozide for Tourette syndrome; in the company's view, the drug was not considered significantly better than Haldol, already on the market. But the Tourette Syndrome Association urged McNeil to undertake a study, and the company agreed to do so. Collins emphasized that FDA regulations and practices in general discourage companies from pursuing orphan applications of marketed drugs. As one example, he cited the current "Good Clinical Practice" regulations of FDA, which, he said, provide clinical investigators and drug sponsors with little opportunity to explore unexpected activities of a drug that are encountered during clinical trials. Additionally, he said, working concurrently on R&D of a secondary use of a drug almost inevitably results in FDA delay in reviewing and approving the drug's primary indication.[32] For these and other reasons, a drug such as pimozide poses problems for drug sponsors. Like haloperidol, pimozide can have serious side effects. Also, only a limited number of patients are available who can be included in clinical trials, and the drug is being tested in a disease whose pathophysiology is not well understood. Yet pimozide was marketed abroad, and U.S. patients wanted an opportunity to see whether it would work for them.

Collin's testimony paled in the glare created by Klugman's, but it emphasized important considerations from a company that had been as responsive as almost any in the orphan-drug area. Similarly, the testimony of Lewis Engman, speaking as president of the PMA, was anticlimactic (most of the television reporters had left) but significant. He announced that the PMA was establishing a Commission on Drugs for Rare Diseases, which would serve as an information clearinghouse to member companies on orphan drugs brought to its attention. In this way, Engman said, the PMA can be certain no useful therapy goes undeveloped for lack of information. Though less than many had hoped for, this was the first public statement by industry on its orphan-drug plans. Engman's message was this: Industry already had been involved in several orphan-drug projects, and it would continue to meet the challenge posed by rare diseases; but FDA should make changes in its regulatory review process, which has increased R&D costs tenfold. Further, he added, FDA should defer to institutional review board approvals for phase I and II clinical studies, rather than monitoring those phases itself, and should use standing advisory committees to resolve scientific disagreements betwen FDA and a drug sponsor. He concluded by urging the FDA to accept foreign data on the same basis as U.S. data. These measures, according to the PMA, would lower costs, stimulating overall research effort and hence development of drugs for rare diseases.[33]

FDA's testimony, presented by J. Richard Crout, provided no similar new announcements, but it reiterated FDA's commitment to efforts to find commercial sponsors and address problems of orphan drugs through regulatory flexibility. Crout described the agency's participation in the Interagency Task Force, its provision of technical assistance for certain drugs sponsored by university scientists, and its capability to modify orphan-drug review processes. He provided a list of drugs of limited commercial value. Some of these had commercial sponsors by dint of FDA efforts and were available on the market; others had commercial sponsors but were not marketed; and some still had no commercial sponsors, indicating more needed to be done to solve the problems.[34]

Although Weiss's bill was never reported out of committee, it had served two vital functions: It had provided a legislative forum for channeling the intense public interest in the issue generated by Klugman's performances in the "Quincy" show and at the Capitol. Moreover, it had precipitated industry's first public statement acknowledging that problems may exist and advancing PMA's suggested remedies.

About two weeks later Representative Robert Kastenmeier (D-Wisc.) introduced H.R. 1937, the Patent Term Restoration Act. The bill sought to amend the patent laws to extend the term of a patent's duration by the period consumed by required regulatory review of a patented product, not to excede seven additional years. Drugs were one of the categories covered under the act.[35] The Office of Technology Assessment (OTA) report on patent term restoration (cited in previous chapters) provided several conclusions about the likely implications of the legislation for drugs intended for small markets. First, the report concluded, patent term extension would increase the attractiveness of research on drugs for large markets but not on those for small markets; therefore, the proposed extension appeared detrimental to research on drugs for rare diseases. The proposed legislation seemed more promising, however, for drugs in other orphan categories, according to the OTA. If the patent term were extended, the OTA staff concluded, more research efforts might be directed toward second uses for existing drugs, including orphan uses. The bill might also result in more research directed toward drugs subject to extensive testing requirements, including those for chronic use and those whose efficacy might be more difficult to establish.[36] The Kastenmeier bill generated enormous controversy because of several of its potential consequences, and congressional efforts to develop an alternative measure succeeded with enactment of a new law in September, 1984 (discussed in chapter 8).

In the meantime, Representative Jamie Whitten (D-Miss.), chairman of the House Appropriations Committee and of its Agriculture, Rural Development, and Related Agencies subcommittee, which has authority over FDA appropriations, took a special interest in orphan drugs. He viewed the term broadly to include not only drugs for rare diseases, but also those that were unpatentable or had other market liabilities that were slowing their introduction in the United States. He was particularly concerned about reports of drugs available in other countries that were not being tested or approved for U.S. marketing. The 1980 General Accounting Office (GAO) report on FDA drug approval, for instance, had found that all but one of fourteen important new drugs had been available in other countries, particularly Switzerland and the United Kingdom, before their U.S. market entry. These included disopyramide for treating abnormal heart rhythm; propranolol for treating high blood pressure; sodium valproate for treating epilepsy; bromocriptine to treat certain endocrine disorders and parkinsonism; and somatotropin to stimulate pituitary growth hormone in children whose growth was prematurely slowed. Moreover, the 1980 GAO report indicated that FDA's formal policy on acceptance of foreign data was not clear.[37] Representative Whitten said that although he was not a scientist, there seemed to be a problem making these drugs available to U.S. citizens, and something needed to be done. He added that since FDA officials supported the current regulatory system, subcommittee staff were asking them and other experts for advice on solving the problem.[38]

On the basis of the forthcoming advice, Whitten decided that FDA should have a means for focusing attention and efforts to deal with problems of orphan drugs. So during 1981 subcommittee hearings on FDA appropriations, Chairman Whitten requested FDA to describe its orphan-drug activities and indicate their current levels of support. FDA officials responded by saying the agency intended to spend $1.5 million out of various budgeted programs in FY 1982 for these activities. Representative Whitten's questions set into motion a structural reorganization at FDA, which created the Office of Orphan Product Development, to be headed by Marion Finkel. The following year, with Representative Whitten's continued commitment to the problem, Congress added $500,000 to FDA's request for $1.5 million specifically for orphan drugs for FY 1983, providing a total of $2 million for activities of the office as well as those undertaken on behalf of orphan drugs in other parts of the agency, including the Center for Drugs, Medical Devices and Biologics, and the National Center for Toxicology, according to Robert McCloud of FDA's budget office.[39] The added $500,000 was to be spent on orphan-drug grants to be awarded by FDA. The agency's FY 1984 budget, according to McCloud, totaled $2.5 million, of which $1 million was earmarked for grants. The projected FY 1985 budget item for the program of $2.6 million requested by FDA was raised by the House to $2.9 million and justified by a congressional determination that a large number of orphan-drug grant requests have not been awarded for lack of funds. Under the House-passed bill, the $2.9 million would include $1.3 million for grants in FY 1985. Thus Representative Whitten achieved the first actual appropriations specifically earmarked for federal funding of orphan-drug projects through grants.

Another approach to the problem was the introduction of H.R. 3260, the proposed Compassionate Drug Availability Act of 1981, by Representative James Scheuer (D-N.Y.), on April 27, 1981. The Scheuer bill, which would have amended the Federal Food Drug and Cosmetic Act (FFDCA), sought to maximize the availability of investigational drugs maintained as Compassionate INDs. Orphan drugs were defined in his bill as those intended to treat diseases or conditions of low incidence—drugs with little projected commercial value because of small numbers of users or lack of exclusive market rights. The act would have authorized such unmarketed drugs for use in patients for diagnostic, treatment, or prevention purposes, but not for clinical trial purposes for benefit/risk assessment; and it would have limited record-keeping requirements solely to case records, and reporting requirements solely to adverse effects. The Scheuer bill also would have allowed such drugs to be exported to other countries requesting them. This was an attempt to deal with the existing problem that drugs that have not gained FDA approval cannot be exported by the United States to other nations.[40] As matters now stand, the export limitation prevents U.S. companies from providing drugs for diseases with rare incidence or prevalence in this country (for which sponsors may not choose to seek FDA approval), to countries where the disease is more common or even endemic. No action was taken on the bill.

All these attempts to deal with various orphan drug problems came to a head on December 15, 1981, when Representative Waxman introduced H.R. 5238, the Orphan Drug Act. As chairman of the Subcommittee on Health and the Environment of the House Committee on Energy and Commerce, Representative Waxman had convened and presided sympathetically over the hearings for both the Holtzman and the Weiss bills. He announced that orphan drugs were a priority issue of the subcommittee, and said he and his subcommittee staff had increased their efforts to explore legislative options.

The Waxman bill contained seven provisions, most of them amending the FFDCA. The first was a statement of need: It called for changes in applicable federal laws to provide for development of drugs for rare diseases, commonly called orphan drugs. The second proposed amending the FFDCA to authorize FDA approval of an orphan drug based on one (instead of the customary two) adequate and well-controlled clinical trial if that trial demonstrated drug efficacy. The third called for amending the FFDCA to authorize FDA to require a rare-disease drug sponsor to maintain data collection on the drug's effectiveness in public use (essentially, postmarket surveillance). The fourth provided for amendment of FFDCA to make drugs for rare diseases still under investigation available to patients for treatment in the absence of any suitable alternative therapy and, at the sponsor's request, to have FDA designate a drug as one for a rare disease, if FDA concurred in that assessment. If so, FDA was to make the drug's designation public. The fifth sought to amend the FFDCA to establish a seven-year period of market exclusivity for unpatentable drugs upon approval by FDA. The sixth called for establishing an interagency committee on orphan-drug development in DHHS, comprising federal employees from agencies involved in drug research and testing. The new committee would be mandated to evaluate and coordinate all government activities on drugs for rare diseases and to promote the development of such drugs. The committee would report annually to Congress. Finally, the seventh proposed amending the Internal Revenue Code to establish a tax credit for a taxable year for any pharmaceutical company developing a drug for a rare disease. The credit would be equal to the amount of research costs during the taxable year attributable to human clinical testing of the drug.[41]

Waxman had decided to limit this legislation specifically to drugs for rare diseases or conditions. Although much concern had been expressed about other problems conferring orphan status, particularly lack of patent protection and greater-than-average liability risks, Representative Waxman concluded that one bill could not accomplish everything. Drugs for rare diseases or conditions constituted a well-defined area and a good starting point. But both he and subcommittee staff, especially counsel William Corr, wanted to become better informed on specific orphan-drug issues and to confirm statements about the problems of orphan drugs that had been made but not documented systematically. During an interview with subcommittee staff (congressional stakeholders) we discussed one means of achieving this purpose. The decision was made to explore market and regulatory factors attending drugs listed by the PMA and FDA provided during the earlier hearings on the Weiss bill. Some drugs listed had commercial sponsors; others did not. Why? Why were some drugs for rare diseases available on the market while others were not? Would approaches included in the legislation help to minimize the differences? The FDA list was entitled "Drugs with Limited Commercial Value." Were these all drugs for rare diseases? Additionally, a GAO study on federal drug development programs requested by Representative Waxman had indicated that the NIH was involved with research on more than 100 drugs.[42] What was the nature of these drug activities of NIH and of the Alcohol, Drug Abuse and Mental Health Administration (ADAMHA) and the Centers for Disease Control (CDC)? Were their problems and needs effectively dealt with in the proposed legislation? Waxman decided to find out in order to help determine which legislative measures would most effectively address realities of the situation as seen by those who knew it best—namely, those directly involved in drug R&D, approval, and distribution. Hearings on H.R. 5238 would be held early in 1982, and Representative Waxman wanted a clearer picture of the situation by then. Subcommittee staff members thereupon immersed themselves in an intense, time-limited orphan-drug survey.

Notes

1. Donald Schön, *Beyond the Stable State* (New York: Basic Books, 1981), pp. 120–125.

2. Bernard Kemp, Appendix to the Interim Report of the Committee on Drugs of Limited Commercial Value, FDA, 1975, unpublished.

3. Interim Report.

4. C.H. Asbury, "Medical Drugs of Limited Commercial Interest: The Development of Federal Policy," Johns Hopkins School of Hygiene and Public Health, 1981, pp. 157–175.

5. *Report of the Commission to Combat Huntingtons Disease and its Consequences* (Bethesda, Md.: NIH, 1976), pp. 1501–1510.

6. Asbury, "Medical Drugs," pp. 180–181.

7. John Adams, PMA, personal communication, 1980.

8. *Significant Drugs of Limited Commercial Value,* Interagency Task Force Report to the Secretary of DHEW (Rockville, Md.: FDA, 1979), pp. 1–82; Marion Finkel, "Drugs of Limited Commercial Value," *New England Journal of Medicine 302*(1980):643–644.

9. C.H. Asbury and Paul Stolley, "Orphan Drugs: Creating a Policy," *Annals of Internal Medicine 95*(2)(1981):221–224.

10. Ibid.

11. C. West Churchman, *The Systems Approach* (New York: Delacorte Press, 1968), pp. 1–227; Russell Ackoff, *A Concept of Corporate Planning* (New York: John Wiley & Sons, 1970); Edward Freeman and David Reed, "Stockholders and Stakeholders: A New Perspective on Corporate Governance," *California Management Review 25*(1983):88–106.

12. Russell Ackoff and Fred Emery, *On Purposeful Systems* (Chicago: Aldine, 1972), pp. 108–109.

13. Roger Battistella and Steven Eastaugh, "Hospital Cost Containment," in Arthur Levin, ed., *Regulating Health Care,* Proceedings of the Academy of Political Science, vol. 33, no. 4, p. 202.

14. Ackoff and Emery, *Purposeful Systems,* pp. 196–207.

15. Government Accounting Office, "FDA Drug Approval—A Lengthy Process That Delays the Availability of Important New Drugs," HRD-80-64, May 28, 1980, p. 30.

16. Gerald Laubach, "Federal Regulation and Pharmaceutical Innovation," in Levin, *Regulating Health Care,* pp. 60–80.

17. Arthur Levin, "The Search for New Forms of Control," in Levin, *Regulating Health Care,* pp. 1–5; Thomas Althius, "Orphan Drugs, Debunking a Myth," *New England Journal of Medicine 303*(17)(1980):1004–1005.

18. C.H. Asbury, "A Systems Approach to Orphan Drugs," Ph.D. dissertation (Ann Arbor: University Microfilms International, 1982), pp. 90–92.

19. Milton Friedman, "Does Business Have a Social Responsibility?" *Bank Administration* (1977).

20. Battistella and Eastaugh, "Hospital Cost Containment," p. 204.

21. Senator Edward Kennedy: "S1075," *Congressional Record*, March 16, 1978.

22. A. Fox, personal communication, 1980.

23. John Adams, PMA, personal communication, 1980.

24. C.H. Asbury, "Medical Drugs of Limited Commercial Interest: Profit Alone is a Bitter Pill," *International Journal of Health Service 11*(3)(1981): 451–462.

25. D. Remer, personal communication, 1980.

26. J. Richard Crout, "New Drug Regulation and Its Impact on Innovation," in S. Mitchell and E. Link, eds., *Impact of Public Policy on Drug Innovation and Pricing* (Washington, D.C.: American University, 1976), pp. 241–317.

27. Representative Elizabeth Holtzman, H.R. 7089, 96th Congress, 2d Session, April 17, 1980.

28. Ross Baldessarini, "Drugs and the Treatment of Psychiatric Disorders," in Alfred Goodman Gilman, Louis Goodman, and Alfred Gilman, eds., *The Pharmacological Basis of Therapeutics*, p. 418.

29. Lilly Engstrom, NIH, Small Business Innovation Research Coordinator, presentation at Cooperative Approaches to Research and Development of Orphan Drugs Meeting, April 10, 1984, Mt. Sinai, New York.

30. Jack Klugman and Adam Seligman, "Statements," *Health and the Environment, Miscellaneous,* Part 2, Hearings, Orphan Drugs, H.R. 1663, March 9, 1981 (Washington, D.C.: U.S. Government Printing Office, Serial No. 97-17, 1981), pp. 10–16.

31. "Leave of Reality," editorial, *Wall Street Journal*, March 12, 1981.

32. David Collins, McNeil, "Statement," Ibid., pp. 136–40.

33. Lewis Engman, PMA, "Statement," Ibid. pp. 73–94.

34. J. Richard Crout, "Statement," Ibid., pp. 24–32.

35. Representative Robert Kastenmeier, H.R. 1937, "Patent Term Restoration Act of 1981," 97th Congress, 1st Session.

36. Office of Technology Assessment, *Patent-Term Extension and the Pharmaceutical Industry* (Washington, D.C.: U.S. Government Printing Office, 1981), pp. 5, 45.

37. GAO report, "FDA," Ibid., pp. 6–8, 42.

38. Representative Jamie Whitten, chairman, House Appropriations Committee, and chairman, Subcommittee on Agriculture, Rural Development, and Related Agencies, personal communication, May 1984.

39. Robert McCloud, FDA Budget Office, personal communication, May 1984.

40. James Scheuer, H.R. 3260, "Compassionate Drug Availability Act of 1981," 97th Congress, 1st Session.

41. Henry Waxman, H.R. 5238, "Orphan Drug Act," 97th Congress, 1st Session.

42. General Accounting Office, *Federal Drug Development Programs* (Washington, D.C.: U.S. General Accounting Office, B-202161, 103964, July 17, 1981).

6
The Orphan Drug Survey

Between December 1981 and February 1982, staff of the House Subcommittee on Health and the Environment carried out a comprehensive survey of the pharmaceutical industry companies and federal agencies concerned with orphan drugs. Survey questions derived in large part from comments made by officials from industry, government, and academia during previous interviews, prior testimony, and lobbying efforts aimed at the earlier bills dealing with orphan-drug problems. Since there had been no joint industry-government planning on orphan drugs, no real dialogue between those with opposing views, and no documentation of characteristics that might help differentiate failed (unsponsored) from successful orphan-drug candidates, the survey appeared to be one mechanism for ascertaining fact and opinion, both of which tend to influence decision making.

As C. West Churchman of Berkeley, one of the developers of the systems approach, had commented, the logical analysis of mathematics at best reveals *how* problems ought to be solved under certain conditions, but not *what* problems ought to be solved. It seemed plausible to Churchman, therefore, that "verification" of research on social systems is the creation of a political process in which opposing groups are more fully aware of each other's world view and of the role of data in the battle for power. Some principles of the systems approach, in Churchman's view, are:

1. It begins when people see the world through the eyes of others.
2. It goes on to discover that every world view is terribly restricted.
3. There are no experts in the systems approach, the public always knows more and the problem is to learn what "everybody" knows.[1]

With this goal in mind, subcommittee staff and this university health policy researcher teamed up to conduct and analyze an orphan-drug survey in late December 1981. The survey covered drugs for rare diseases or conditions identified by industry sponsors, and drugs in which federal agencies were involved. The survey was completed within weeks, with full cooperation by pharmaceutical firms and federal agencies. Data obtained, though preliminary and descriptive, did reveal some patterns meriting additional study. Even in preliminary stages of analysis, as Representative Waxman later remarked at the hearing on the Orphan Drug Act, the survey helped to confirm and define problems that had been described as barriers to development by commercial drug sponsors, and to suggest that there were market and regulatory factors that could be changed beneficially through legislation.

Survey Methods

Drugs surveyed were those contained in three lists. One was the PMA list of 72 drugs for rare diseases and conditions sponsored by industry and available on the market or in Compassionate IND status. A second was the list developed by the 1978 Interagency Task Force on Drugs of Limited Commercial Value, presented at the Weiss bill hearings, and later updated by FDA at Representative Douglas Walgren's (D-Penna.) request. The additional list, entitled "Drugs of Limited Commercial Value for Which No or Little Marketing Interest Has Been Shown," included 32 drugs. The third was an expansion and revision, under the direction of subcommittee staff counsel William Corr, of the list generated by the General Accounting Office (GAO) of drugs in which federal agencies were involved. Drugs of the Department of Defense, listed by the GAO, were not included because they were considered to be intended for special cases—for use in wartime or in specific geographic areas. Subcommittee staff expanded the GAO list to include drugs from CDC and ADAMHA as well as NIH. A total of 290 drugs was identified by all federal research agencies, and the grand total from all sources was 394 drugs.

Because severe time limitations precluded surveying all 394 drugs, a stratified random sample was taken instead. A 100 percent sample was taken of PMA- and FDA-identified drugs, and a 32 percent sample was taken of drugs identified by federal research agencies on the basis that the former two had included drugs specifically considered orphan or of little commercial value, whereas the criteria for federal agency listings was simply involvement with the drugs. In all, 196 drugs were surveyed. Each questionnaire concerned only one drug, and only one view per drug was sought. Therefore, if a drug initially had been developed by government researchers but was included on the PMA list as being sponsored currently by a PMA member firm, only the drug's commercial sponsor was asked to fill out the questionnaire. This may have depleted the richness of aggregate views on any one drug, but staff had decided that to send out more than one questionnaire per drug might jeopardize the spirit of trust characterizing the survey effort.

Since federally identified drugs were not confined to those for rare conditions or diseases, federal agency respondents were provided with both an orphan and a nonorphan questionnaire version for each drug. The respondent was to determine whether the drug was for a rare disease or condition, and then to provide the estimated population size, rather than having the subcommittee impose a definition of *rare*. Industry sponsors received only the orphan-drug questionnaire version, since use in a rare disease or condition was the criterion according to which drugs were included in the PMA list; industry respondents also were asked to provide the estimated population size for the drug. Through this method, the subcommittee sought a general consensus delimiting the term *rare* by those involved in drug development.

Subcommittee staff were less concerned with comparing characteristics of federally identified drugs to their industrially sponsored counterparts than with grasping the nature and extent of federal drug activities. This limited the ability to compare and contrast federal- and industry-identified drugs, except in very general, descriptive terms. Nonetheless, in the absence of any systematic description of federal drug R&D efforts, this appeared to be a necessary first step. Complicating comparison further was the need to include the option of a "don't know" answer to many of the questions posed to federal drug sponsors. Rarely was this option provided to industry sponsors, who were expected to know the specifics of market and regulatory characteristics of drugs. This turned out to be a widely used option by federal respondents, who in many instances knew very little about such factors as patent status, development costs, and liability problems. In one instance, where a federal sponsor of several drugs had checked the "don't know" option wherever offered, the person coding the questionnaires was prompted to ask whether the respondent actually worked at NIH or was just renting a room there.

The high percentage of "don't know" responses may have resulted from a problem in conveying the subcommittee's purposes to those in federal agencies actually filling out the questionnaire. Prior to sending questionnaires, members of the PMA commission, as well as officials of CDC, NIH, and FDA, had been asked to review them; to make suggestions on any questions that were considered unclear, ambiguous, or too invasive; and to identify important issues that were not addressed. Useful comments from all these sources were provided to the subcommittee staff, and questionnaires were amended accordingly. Those who reviewed questionnaires, however, often were not those who ultimately answered them. Moreover, it appears that the covering letter from Representative Waxman, explaining the nature of the survey, was not transmitted to these individual federal agency respondents. As one government researcher put it, he thought he was entering a damned-if-you-do, damned-if-you-don't situation—open to criticism for failing to seek industry assistance and therefore spending taxpayer dollars on drugs industry might develop; or, conversely, for being in collusion with industry on joint development projects. Criticism for either situation was not the subcommittee's intent, but the message was garbled in transmission through bureaucratic channels.

Industry sponsors, on the other hand, each received a letter explaining the survey's purposes and requesting participation. Although it may be argued that data by subpoena (a tongue-in-cheek reference to the command power of the subcommittee) has a decided advantage in stimulating survey participation, industry comments appeared to be straightforward, informative, and extremely useful in presenting a view of each drug's specific problems. PMA commission members made it known to member firms that they had been consulted on the survey and in general supported the subcommittee's information efforts, and this too probably helped to enrich industry participation. There was a 100 percent response rate from both industry and government.

Finally, all respondents were asked to indicate whether the orphan drug was developed for the orphan indication first (or solely), or secondarily to a nonorphan use. Many characteristics of the drugs then could be viewed with this distinction in mind.

Survey Results

Of the 196 drugs surveyed, sponsors considered 134 to be for use in rare diseases or conditions, as shown in Table 6–1, which was included in the subcommittee report.[2] Thirteen of these drugs sponsored by federal agency scientists, however, were judged to be in too early a stage of development for scientists to assess potential therapeutic benefit. The current analysis excludes these drugs.

On the basis of the survey, industry was sponsoring 58 orphan drugs for rare diseases or conditions; 34 of these were available on

Table 6–1
Drugs Surveyed by Questionnaire

Respondents	Question-naires Sent	Additional Question-naires Returned[a]	Drugs Considered Nonorphan by Respondent[b]	Drugs Considered Orphan by Respondent
Industry				
(26 firms)[c]	72	4	18	58
ADAMHA	25	—	17	8
NIH	58	—	22	36
CDC	15	1	—	16
FDA	23	—	10[d]	13
Private				
researchers	3	—	—	13
Totals	196	5	67	134[e]

[a]Additional drugs identified by sponsors as orphan.

[b]Not for rare disease, or are research tools.

[c]Four of these firms indicated they had no orphan drugs.

[d]Four of these drugs were considered nonorphan; six had commercial sponsors, so FDA did not complete questionnaires on them.

[e]Total of column 1 + column 2 minus column 3 = total of column 4.

the market, and 24 were in Compassionate IND status, as shown in Tables 6–2 and 6–3. On the basis of the survey sample, an additional 228 drugs or biologicals intended for use in rare disorders were under study by federal research agency scientists or grantees. If one included drugs that were in too early an investigational stage for scientists to assess likely use in orphan diseases, the total could have reached 295 orphan drugs. Moreover, if drugs were included that were deemed by federal agency scientists to be of little commercial interest based on factors other than population size (such as vaccines and contraceptives) the total may have risen to 344 drugs. Finally, since the FDA list was not based on an exhaustive search of drugs sponsored by academic scientists, this segment of orphan-drug activity may be underrepresented.[3] Because data from pharmaceutical industry sponsors are the most inclusive, they receive the most emphasis.

Market Factors

A certain number of the industrially sponsored drugs in Compassionate IND status are probably there as a matter of timing. For instance, at the time of the survey, 7 of these drugs had NDA ap-

Table 6–2
Marketed Drugs Sponsored by PMA Member Firms

Sponsor	Drug	Condition
Hoffmann–LaRoche	Ancoban (flucytosine)	Systemic candida or cryptococcus infection
	Clonopin (clonazepam)	Minor motor seizures, myoclonic seizures
	FUDR (floxuridine)	Anticancer agent infused regionally
	Rocaltrol (calcitriol)	Hypocalcemia; chronic renal dialysis
	Solatene (beta carotene)	Erythropoietic protoporphyria
	Bactrim (sulfmethoxazole-trimethoprim	Pneumocystis
Norwich Eaton Pharmaceuticals	Dantrium Intravenous (dantrolene)	Malignant hyperthermia crisis
Bristol	Lysodren (mitotane)	Inoperable adrenal carcinoma
Merck & Co., Inc.	Elspar (asparaginase)	Acute lymphocytic leukemia
	Demser (metyrosine)	Chronic or preoperative malignant pheochromocytoma
Sandoz	Parlodel (bromocriptine)	Acromegaly
	Diapid (lypressin)	Endogenous antidiuretic hormone deficiency
Cutter Laboratories	Plague Vaccine	Active immunization
	Rabies Immune Globulin	Passive immunization
Burroughs Wellcome Co.	Injectable Imuran (azothioprine)	Rejection prevention in renal homotransplantation
	Myleran (busulfan)	Chronic granulocytic leukemia
	Thioguanine	Acute myeloblastic leukemia of childhood
A.H. Robins Company	Reglan Injectable (metaclopramide)	Diabetic gastroparesis
Schering-Plough Corporation	Proglycem (diazoxide)	Hypoglycemia
	Hyperstat I.V. (diazoxide)	Malignant hypertension
Ciba-Geigy Corporation	Cytadren	Cushings syndrome
	Desferal (deferoxamine)	Thalassemia
Miles Pharmaceuticals	Mithromycin (mithracin)	Testicular malignant tumors
	DTIC (dacarbazine)	Metastatic malignant melanoma
Alcon Laboratories	Natacyin (natamycin)	Ophthalmic fungal infections
Abbott Laboratories	Depakene (valproic acid)	Absence seizures
	Cylert (pemoline)	Hyperkinetic syndrome
	Relefact TRH (protirelin)	Adjunctive diagnostic agent (pituitary, thyroid dysfunction)
Ayerst Laboratories	Peptavlon (pentagastrin)	Diagnostic (gastric acid secretion)
	Protopam Chloride	Poison antidote; anticholinesterase overdose control

Table 6–2

Sponsor	Drug	Condition
The Upjohn Company	Calderol	Metabolic bone disease associated with chronic renal failure
	Prostin VR	Pre-surgical palliation of ductus arteriosus
Winthrop Laboratories	Danocrine	Hereditary angioneurotic edema
Pfizer Inc.	Mithracin	Testicular cancer

plications filed with FDA; the review had not been completed when the survey was made. The remaining 17 drugs appeared to be in indefinite Compassionate IND status. Sponsors of 7 of these drugs said they intended to file NDA applications although the drugs have been under development for longer than is the norm; sponsors of 5 drugs were undecided, and sponsors of the remaining 5 drugs did not intend to seek marketing approval. Four of these last drugs are for conditions affecting fewer than 1,000 people in the United States.[4]

Introduction of orphan-drug INDs has remained relatively constant since 1962. The average was about 2 drugs per year, with the exception of an initial spurt in 1963, just after the 1962 Kefauver-Harris amendments to the Food, Drug and Cosmetic Act were being implemented by FDA, which now required drug sponsors to submit INDs. A total of 17 PMA member companies have sponsored an average of two marketed orphan drugs each since 1962, as shown in Table 6–4. When including both marketed and Compassionate IND drugs, a total of 22 companies have sponsored an average of 2.6 orphan drugs each, ranging from 1 to 10 drugs per firm.

Most orphan drugs identified by industry and federal agency sponsors are intended for U.S. populations of fewer than 100,000 persons, as shown in Table 6–5. In fact, 75 percent of industry and of federally sponsored drugs are intended for 50,000 or fewer people in the United States. Nonetheless, 12 percent of industry drugs and close to 20 percent of federally identified drugs considered orphan were intended for use by from 100,000 to more than 1 million people. This suggests that federal researchers' perceptions of small market may be more conservative than those of the industry in general, and that the range of population size considered orphan makes any designated cutoff limit subject to special case considerations.

Some general features can be gleaned from the data. For instance, industry-sponsored drugs tend to be for chronic or short-term use as opposed to single administration. Many have nonorphan uses. Slightly more than two-fifths (42 percent) are the sole drug therapy available

Table 6–3
Compassionate IND Drugs Sponsored by PMA Member Firms[a]

Sponsor	Drug	Condition
Hoffmann–LaRoche	Mogadon (nitrazepam)	Anticonvulsant, infantile spasms
	Pyridostigmine Chloride	Myasthenia gravis
	Nitoman (tetrabenazine)	Huntingtons disease, movement disorders
	Thymosin	Congenital immunodeficiencies
Bristol	Teniposide	Refractory pediatric neuroblastoma
McNeil Pharmaceutical	SEMAP (penfluridol)	Tourette syndrome
	ORAP (pimozide)	Tourette syndrome
	ORAP (pimozide)	Monosymptomatic hypochondriacal psychosis
	ORAP (pimozide)	Generalized lipodystrophy
Burroughs Wellcome Co.	Zyloprim Injectable (allopurinol)	Hyperuricemia in cancer therapy
The Upjohn Company	Zanosar (streptozotocin)	Metastatic pancreatic islet cell carcinoma
	Mylosae	Acute myelogenous leukemia
Eli Lilly and Company	Frentizole	Idiopathic thrombocytopenia purpura
Knoll Pharmaceutical Company	Isoptin (verapamil)	Idiopathic hypertrophic subaortic stenosis
Winthrop Laboratories	Trilostane	Cushings syndrome
	Trilostane	Conns syndrome
	Danocrine (danazol)	Precocious puberty
Pfizer Inc.	Fenclonine P.O.	Carcinoid syndrome
	Mithracin I.V.	Pagets disease
SmithKline Beckman Laboratories	Cytomel Injectable (liothyronine)	Myxedema coma
Ciba-Geigy	Cibacalcin	Pagets disease
Company Sponsorships That Are Confidential	3 Drugs	Names of drugs and corporate sponsors confidential[b]

[a]As of February 1981; some of these drugs now may be approved and on the market.
[b]Drugs not listed in "Results of Survey on Orphan Drugs" prepared by the PMA, on which the Waxman survey was based. Responses on these three drugs provided by sponsoring companies.

for the intended disease or condition. Drugs tend to be for neoplastic (13 drugs), endocrine (11 drugs) or neurologic disorders (8 drugs). There were from 1 to 5 drugs in other categories, including psychiatric, drug abuse, vaccines, anti-infectives, cardiocirculatory, metabolic, hematologic, physiological tools, or miscellaneous, as grouped either by organ system or by general usage. Generally their development costs were about average compared to those for other drugs developed by companies responding. Slightly more than two-thirds of the industry-sponsored marketed orphan drugs had federal or uni-

Table 6–4

Marketed Orphan Drugs Identified by Industry, Number per Sponsor

Drugs per Firm	Number of Firms	Percentage of Firms	Total Drugs
1	6	35	6
2	8	47	16
3	2	12	6
6	1	6	6
Total	17	100	34

Table 6–5

Estimated Orphan Market Size (or Pool of Users) by Drug Status and by Sponsor

Estimated Number of U.S. Patients to be Treated per Annum	Industry Drugs (%)			Federal Drugs (%)	
	Marketed Drugs	Compassionate INDs[a]	Compassionate INDs[b]	NDAs	INDs
Under 10,000	50	43	76	20	65
Under 50,000	73.5	43	92	50	80
Under 100,000	82	86	100	50	84

[a]Compassionate INDs with NDA's pending.

[b]Compassionate INDs in that status indefinitely.

versity assistance. Liability suits had been filed for nearly one-fifth (18 percent) of marketed orphan drugs, suggesting legal concerns are not unfounded. Since no data are available on the percentage of suits filed against manufacturers for drugs in general, however, no conclusions can be drawn about whether orphan drugs pose unusually high liability risks. Foreign data were available at the time the IND was filed for nearly two-fifths of industry-identified drugs, suggesting that U.S. orphan-drug development may lag behind efforts in other countries. Finally, industry-identified drugs, especially those developed recently, tend to be protected by patent. Many of these points and some others are next discussed more fully.

Nearly one-half (45 percent) of industry-sponsored orphan drugs have nonorphan uses. Of the 34 marketed drugs, 8 initially were developed for use in common diseases or conditions and subsequently were found to have orphan uses. The extent of orphan uses of nonorphan drugs in general is not known; but, 7, or one out of every 3.7 of the remaining 26 marketed orphan drugs initially developed for an orphan indication, later was found to have a nonor-phan indication as well. These are instances of commercial losers converting to commercial contenders, if not outright winners, at a rate of about 30 percent of the total—a fact to be kept in mind when considering orphan-drug policy. The good odds of finding common-disease uses for these drugs make them a compelling market gamble.

Three-quarters of orphan drugs in indefinite Compassionate IND status also have applications pending for nonorphan uses. But some of these nonorphan NDA applications have been under FDA review for as long as nine years, and some sponsors said they were awaiting FDA nonorphan decisions before deciding whether to file supple-mental NDAs for the drugs' orphan indications. Most indefinite Compassionate INDs are for use in chronic disease, and for all but 2 of the 15 drugs on which information was provided, alternative drugs were available. Therefore, data suggest that prolonged use of the Compassionate IND mechanism occurs with drugs that have difficult safety and efficacy reviews, or those that are intended for minute numbers of patients.[5]

Ten of the 34 marketed orphan drugs were developed solely by the companies responding, with no federal or university assistance. Government or university participation in developing the remaining 24 drugs consisted primarily of conducting clinical trials. This may reflect a general industry practice of involving academic or federally supported research clinicians in clinical trials generally, whether for orphan or nonorphan drugs, but the current data do not allow for a comparison. However, they do suggest federal and university sci-entists are asked to take a major role in testing orphan drugs; and, whether for reasons of access to patients, expertise, or economics, it appears that the percentage of orphan drugs under development solely by industry is declining, whereas that for joint industry-government development is increasing. For instance, 86 percent of drugs in Compassionate IND status were jointly developed by in-dustry and government; the median year in which INDs on these drugs were filed was fairly recent, 1975. This contrasts with joint development of only 50 percent of marketed orphan drugs developed solely or initially for an orphan disease; here, the median year for which IND filing took place was ten years earlier, 1965. Although these figures suggest a trend toward greater federal and academic involvement in orphan-drug undertakings by industry, additional information would be needed to draw firm conclusions.

Industry-identified orphan drugs currently on the market took an average of 5.75 years to develop (from the filing of the IND to filing of the NDA). As Table 6–6 indicates, drugs secondarily developed for the orphan indication, and those developed more recently (Compassionate INDs with NDA applications pending) have taken longer to develop than their earlier, marketed counterparts. Total development time (period between IND filing and NDA approval) averaged 7.6 years; that is within the range of the average for all new chemical entities (NCEs) developed in the late 1970s, according to data provided by the FDA to the Office of Technology Assessment (OTA), as shown in Table 6–7. The comparison is limited, however, since many orphan drugs were developed in the 1960s and early 1970s, whereas FDA data concern more recently developed drugs, and total development time has tended to increase in these later years, as the table shows.

Finally, development time for drugs in indefinite Compassionate IND status (excluding those whose sponsors do not intend to submit NDA applications) is substantially longer on average (8.5 years at the time the survey was taken) than that for orphan drugs on the market (5.75 years, exclusive of FDA review time). This suggests development of these drugs is more time-consuming, whether due to technical difficulties or a less-than-vigorous pursuit of approval by sponsors. As noted earlier, sponsors of some of these drugs are awaiting FDA approval decisions on the drug's nonorphan use.

Development costs for industry-sponsored orphan drugs were estimates relative to the average for companies responding. There-

Table 6–6
Development Time of Orphan Drugs Sponsored by Industry
(Period between IND and NDA Filing, in Years)

	Marketed Drugs			Compassionate INDs with NDAs Pending
	1[a]	2[b]	3[c]	
Development (in years)				
Mean	5.3	7	5.8	6.9
Median	5	6.5	5	8
Range	1–10	2–13	1–13	2–10

[a]Developed for orphan indication first.
[b]Developed for orphan indication secondarily.
[c]Aggregate marketed orphan drugs.

Table 6–7
Comparison of Total Development Time
(IND Filed to NDA Approved, in Years)

	Orphan Drugs and All NCE's	
	Mean	*Median*
Orphan drugs (1962–1978)	7.6	7
All NCEs:		
1976	5.8	5
1977	7.8	7
1978	5.2	5
1979	8.9	9
1980	8.2	7.5

Source: Adapted in part from Office of Technology Assessment, *Patent Term Extension and the Pharmaceutical Industry* (Washington, D.C.: U.S. Government Printing Office, 1981), OTA-CIT-143, p. 34.

Table 6–8
Relative Estimated Development Costs by Development Arrangements
$(N = 34)$[a]

Drugs developed by	Less Than Average Cost	Average or Greater Cost
Company alone	5	12
Company and other(s)	12	5

[a]Includes marketed and Compassionate IND drugs sponsored by industry with the exception of the following drugs: those developed prior to the 1962 Kefauver-Harris amendments $(N = 3)$; those whose relative development costs were not known $(N = 3)$; drugs developed by firms other than the one responding or by federal agencies $(N = 13)$; and drugs in Compassionate IND status whose sponsors do not intend to submit NDA applications $(N = 5)$.

fore, data are soft, based on perceptions of both orphan and average drug costs per firm. Such perceptions, however, may influence decisions and provide a perspective on the cost issue in general. Data indicate drugs estimated to cost less than average tended to have had university or federal agency assistance, as shown in Table 6–8. Such assistance was not a guarantee of lower costs, however; two-thirds of drugs had assistance, but fewer than two-fifths had lower than average costs.

As Table 6–9 indicates, a higher percentage of orphan drugs developed in the 1960s have relatively low costs than of those developed in the 1970s. This may reflect higher costs for all drug

Table 6–9
Relative Estimated Development Costs, Industry-
Sponsored Drugs[a] by Decade IND Filed

Estimated Costs	1960s	1970s	Total
Less	8 (40%)	6 (19%)	14
Average	9	21	30
More	3	4	7
Total	20	31	51

[a]Estimates were not provided for drugs developed by companies other than those responding or for those developed by federal agencies whose products were adopted by the firm responding.

Table 6–10
Relative Estimated Development Costs by Whether Drugs
Had Nonorphan Indication

Estimated Relative Development Costs	Total Drugs	Drugs with Nonorphan Uses	Drugs with Orphan Uses Only
Less	14	5	9
Average	30	15	15
More	7	3	4

development, or it may reflect differences in recollections of costs of drugs developed some time ago. It does not appear to be influenced substantially by whether or not the drug was developed for both an orphan and a nonorphan indication (Table 6–10), although drugs costing less to develop tended to be those having only an orphan indication. The perception that only 19 percent of orphan drugs have lower than average costs may suggest that this is an important market barrier according to drug sponsors, especially when 12 percent of drugs were reported to have greater than average development costs, which could be construed as a substantial disincentive. This is especially telling when compared with perceptions of return on investment (ROI). Two-thirds of drug sponsors provided ROI estimates (among sponsors not responding to this question were those whose firms had not developed the drug and those who had substantial federal and academic assistance). ROI was considered less than average for 19 drugs and average for 4. These perceptions are substantiated in part by hard data provided by Thomas Althius of Pfizer.[6] From a comparison of his listing of 1979 Annual Drugstore and Hospital Drug Sales with the PMA list of marketed orphan drugs,

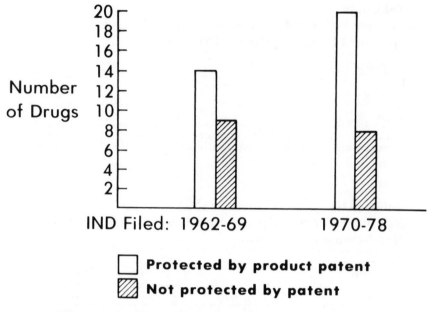

Figure 6–1. Patent Protection by Decade IND Filed

26 percent of these industry-sponsored orphan drugs had sales of less than $1 million, whereas a total of 44 percent of orphan drugs had sales reported to be less than $3 million.

Industry orphan drugs tended to be protected by patent, especially those developed in the 1970s as opposed to the 1960s (see Figure 6–1). Nearly two-thirds had product patents at the time the IND was filed (Table 6–11). Moreover, nonpatentable products tended to be for minute populations, and three of the unpatentable drugs were developed by federal agencies and adopted by pharmaceutical company sponsors. Nevertheless, data show that companies have been willing to develop or sponsor unpatentable drugs, although the trend

Table 6–11
Patent Status,[a] Industry-Sponsored Orphan Drugs

Protected by	Total (%)	Marketed (%)	Compassionate INDs (%)
Product Patent	62.5	53	75
Use Patent Only	12.5	19	4
No Patent	25	28	21

[a]Status at time IND filed.

seems increasingly to favor involvement with those having market protection.

Relative retail costs to the consumer for marketed orphan drugs reportedly are greater than average for more than one-half of such drugs (59 percent). This appears to be correlated with higher than average distribution costs, suggesting these costs are being passed on to consumers or, in cases of consumers' high medical bills, to their health insurers.

Finally, sponsors of fewer than one-half of drugs felt development of orphan products conferred public relations benefits on the company. Successes generally were lifesaving drugs; preventive drugs and biologicals were not public relations assets, according to sponsors. This tends to support the statement by many industry officials who said the PMA had not done enough to publicize orphan-drug activities of member firms.

Regulatory Factors

FDA safety and efficacy guidelines were considered unclear or unavailable to industry by sponsors of about one-half of the orphan drugs. About 44 percent of sponsors said safety guidelines were less clear, on average, than those for other drugs developed by their companies. Some sponsors said no guidelines had been provided. Efficacy guidelines were judged to be less clear than the average by 57 percent of sponsors. Moreover, a number of respondents who considered orphan-drug guidelines to be on a par with those for other drugs said guidelines in general were unclear; those for orphan drugs were no worse than others. Some respondents wrote that variations existed not only between FDA divisions but within them as well.

Four-fifths of sponsors whose drugs were developed initially or solely for orphan uses did not find that the guidelines were a good indication of data actually required by FDA for NDA approval. This lent substantial credibility to industry requests, made during redrafting of the Waxman bill, that the legislation require FDA to provide an assessment to orphan-drug IND holders of likely NDA requirements before sponsors embarked on human trials. In contrast, sponsors of drugs requiring only a supplemental NDA (those drugs developed secondarily for an orphan indication) considered FDA guidelines to be a relatively good indication of actual approvement requirements, suggesting review of second indications holds few surprises.

Two-thirds of industry sponsors felt FDA communicated difficulties about data promptly, and 83 percent said FDA assistance was average or better. Even so, for 80 percent of industry sponsors, clinical trials posed problems—especially in obtaining participants and co-ordinating studies. More than a third of sponsors requested special FDA review considerations, usually for reduced clinical-trial requirements.

FDA review of orphan drugs now on the market took an average of 1.9 years. Reviews are now faster, averaging 1.5 years for NDAs approved during 1975–1981, compared to an average of 2 years for approvals made during 1962–1969. Sponsors confirmed that FDA review periods for 90 percent of drugs were average or less, but many felt the average itself was longer than necessary. Nearly one-quarter (24 percent) of the orphan drugs were reviewed within the 180 day period stipulated by law. This suggests that development problems, rather than delays in NDA review, are the major deterents to relatively rapid orphan-drug availability, and that increased attention should be paid to clarifying guidelines and agreeing on likely requirements to expedite preparation of the NDA.

Finally, the Compassionate IND mechanism received mixed reviews. More than three-quarters of those who have sponsored Compassionate IND drugs considered the mechanism ineffective and particularly inefficient. Slightly more than half of the sponsors said they would prefer another mechanism be developed to serve the purpose of making experimental drugs available to clinicians and researchers. Physician requests for Compassionate INDs ranged from 0.2 to 40 per drug per year for supplies to treat their patients. All these requests require data-gathering and informed-consent processes.

Results from Federal Agency Questionnaires

Generalizations about federally identified drugs are limited. This stems from a number of factors, including diversity of federal programs and difficulties in designing questionnaires to cover the number of variations in types of drugs and drug programs sponsored by federal agencies; difficulties on the part of some institutes (especially the National Heart, Lung and Blood Institute) in identifying drug-related projects; and lack of information on the part of drug sponsors on specific regulatory and market characteristics of drugs.

Perhaps the most significant finding in terms of planning for orphan drugs was the need by agencies to develop improved means of identifying potential drug candidates so that earlier coordination with FDA could be undertaken to ensure that data collected under NIH and ADAMHA drug development grants and contracts are consistent with FDA review requirements. This would provide a means to head off prospectively any major regulatory complications. Another finding was that patent status of about 40 percent of federally-identified drugs was not known. This estimate may be high because patent status of NCI drugs—which comprise a substantial component of federally-identified drugs—was known. Nonetheless in view of the importance of this variable in securing commercial sponsors, it appears that other institutes would do well to obtain at least patent, if not other market information early in development to facilitate the process of transforming these R&D projects into marketed products.

Despite lacks in aggregate data, survey responses provide useful generalizations about the diversity of roles the government assumes on behalf of orphan drugs. The survey sample suggests that about 75 percent of federally identified drugs are for populations of fewer than 50,000 people in the United States. In sum, 80 percent of federally identified drugs were considered to be for orphan indications. Nonorphan categories primarily included vaccines, birth control agents, anti-infectives, cardiocirculatory, and psychiatric drugs. Clinical-testing problems occurred with about one-half of drugs sponsored by federal research agencies.

By far the most extensive drug program is that sponsored by the National Cancer Institute (NCI), as shown in Table 6–12. NCI drugs, stratified in the sample according to development arrangements, tend to be for cancers affecting between 5,000 and 50,000 people, although 17 percent of NCI's orphan drugs were treatments for cancers affecting from 100,000 to 500,000 people in this country. Based on the sample, about two-fifths (41 percent) of drugs were developed jointly by NCI and industry; one-third were developed by NCI alone. Fewer than 10 percent were developed primarily by pharmaceutical sponsors, with NCI participation late in the drugs' development. Most are intended for short-term use, none have nonorphan indications, few have foreign data available, and slightly fewer than one-half of those whose patent status was known were protected by product patents. Small market was cited by federal sponsors as a major disincentive for commercial development; difficulties in safety and particularly efficacy demonstration also were considered market obstacles. Even so, owing to the strong NCI program described in Chapter 3, 25 percent of drugs studied by NCI are on the market, sponsored by industry firms, or are undergoing NDA review by FDA. The rest are still in IND status, currently undergoing studies.

Table 6–12
Federally Identified Drugs,[a] by Agency and Institute

Agency	IND Status	NDA Status	Total
FDA	32	—	32
CDC	20	6	26
ADAMHA:			
NIMH	49	—	49
NIAAA[b]	2	—	2
NIDA	9	1	10
NIH:			
NCI	89	30	119
NIAID	26	14	40
NINCDS	33	5	38
NICHD	5	—	5
NEI[c]	1	—	1
Total	266	56	322

[a]Defined as drugs in which the agencies are involved; these were found to include drugs being used as research tools, and drugs that were in too early a stage of development to assess whether they had therapeutic potential.

[b]National Institute on Alcohol and Alcohol Abuse.

[c]National Eye Institute. The other institutes are identified in the text and the glossary.

The National Institute of Allergy and Infectious Diseases (NIAID) is working primarily with vaccines and anti-infectives. Almost three-fifths are considered orphan drugs or biologicals, intended for fewer than 50,000 people. Those considered nonorphan were for treatment or prevention of disease in 1 million or more people here. These are for short-term or single administration, whereas those drugs and biologicals considered orphan tend also to be for short-term use or for chronic administration. Most have had triangular development by NIAID, university, and industry scientists. Patent status is not known; but one-third of the drugs are on the market or under NDA review, and these tend to have commercial sponsors.

Nearly two-fifths of drugs identified by the National Institute of Mental Health (NIMH) are used as research tools or are in too early a stage of development to assess possible therapeutic use. Of the remaining NIMH drugs, one-half are considered orphan, but with wide variation in the definition. Orphan drugs are intended to treat illnesses ranging from those affecting 1,000 to more than 1 million people in the United States. NIMH has developed about one-half of its drugs for use in treating specific subsets of patients with rare forms of more common illnesses. The institute is testing the remaining drugs to assess more accurately their efficacy in treating common psychiatric disorders. Patent status of drugs generally was not known.

All drugs identified by the National Institute of Neurological and Communicative Disorders and Stroke (NINCDS) were for orphan indications, but more than three-quarters were in too early a stage of development for sponsors to assess their potential usefulness. The other drugs have been developed to treat diseases affecting more than 100,000 but fewer than 500,000 people in this country. They are for chronic use. Some have been developed solely by the institute; others represent joint efforts with industry or academia. Five drugs are on the market. Sponsors of the INDs rarely knew patent status of the drugs.

Although 60 percent of drugs identified by the National Institute on Drug Abuse (NIDA) are used as research tools or are not developed enough to assess potential use, the remaining drugs all are considered orphan. NIDA scientists' definitions of orphan drugs, like those of NIMH scientists, however, cover a wide range. NIDA's orphan drugs include those for treating substance dependencies in as few as 1,000 to 5,000 people, as well as those affecting 1 million or more people in the United States. Drugs tend to have patent protection, and one-half have common as well as orphan uses. Foreign data rarely are available for the drugs, most of which are intended to treat opiate or narcotic addiction or dependence. NIDA alone developed one drug in the survey sample, and collaborated with academia and industry on the rest.

All five drugs identified by the National Institute of Child Health and Human Development (NICHD) are contraceptive agents considered nonorphan, for chronic use, most by more than 1 million people. NICHD respondents cited reasons for industry's perceived lack of interest, including the drugs' high product liability and development costs, and the extended animal safety testing required. Slightly more than half of the agents have product patent protection.

Nearly three-quarters of drugs identified by FDA are considered orphan; most are for treating, preventing, or diagnosing disorders affecting relatively minute numbers of people—about 5,000—in the United States. Most are for chronic or short-term use and have been developed by academic scientists; and only one also has a nonorphan indication. Patent status rarely was known. Many are available as Compassionate INDs. Several are diagnostic or preventive drugs; others provide cures. FDA provided no specific assistance for about half of the drugs, but did assist in protocol development for more than one-third. Additionally, in a few instances FDA assembled data, provided NDA submission assistance or solicited the NDA, or (in two cases) sought a manufacturer. About one-quarter of the drugs identified by FDA were considered nonorphan because they were for use in disorders affecting 500,000 or more people in this country. Still, they lacked commercial sponsors. They are all for chronic use, have federal research or academic scientists as IND sponsors, tend not to be patentable, and are preventive and/or lifesaving. Foreign data are available for at least one-half, suggesting these may be instances of "drug lag" by pharmaceutical companies uninterested in securing NDA approval for use in the United States.

Finally, Centers for Disease Control (CDC) scientists considered all CDC's drugs to be orphan. Most are deemed lifesaving, either curative or preventive antiparasitics or vaccines, intended for short-term and single administration, respectively. CDC has developed a majority of the drugs for use in this country, obtaining drug supplies from foreign firms, most of which market the drugs in countries where the diseases or conditions are more prevalent. Some biologicals have been provided by state health departments. None have nonorphan uses, and none whose patent status was known (about two-thirds) were protected by patent. CDC, which conducts surveillance on infectious disease and monitors use of these specialized biologicals, receives several thousand requests yearly for a few of the biologicals, but most are sought far less frequently.

In sum, the multifaceted federal role is dominated in numbers of drugs and biologicals by programs of NCI, NIAID, and CDC. Characteristics of other drug groups, such as those sponsored by NICHD, NINCDS, and NIMH, may be dwarfed in an aggregate view. Clearly, however, the government is involved in every step of drug R&D and distribution, both alone and in concert with industry. Although projects and programs tend to emphasize drugs and biologicals for rare disorders, the government also is a significant presence in developing drugs for more prevalent conditions, most notably for many cancers, for substance abuse and infectious diseases, and for contraception. Liability risks and lack of market protection attending these drugs for more common conditions appear to have left them as orphans, nurtured by government, despite their potentially large market.

Notes

1. C. West Churchman, *The Systems Approach* (New York: Dell, 1979).

2. *Preliminary Report of the Survey on Drugs for Rare Disease* (Washington, D.C.: U.S. Government Printing Office, 1982), p. 3.

3. *Summary Report of the Survey on Drugs for Rare Disease*, available from the subcommittee.

4. C.H. Asbury, *A Systems Approach to Orphan Drugs* (Ann Arbor: University Microfilms International, 1982), pp. 291–298.

5. Ibid., p. 292.

6. Thomas Althius, "Contributions of the Pharmaceutical Industry," in Fred Karch, ed., *Orphan Drugs* (New York: Marcel Dekker, 1982), pp. 185–187.

7
Enactment of the Orphan Drug Law

T he orphan-drug survey defined more clearly the issues addressed in H.R. 5238, the Orphan Drug Act, which were then discussed during the March 1982 hearings on the bill. Thereafter, the process of crafting the final legislative version took place in the real world of posturing and maneuvering, compromise and conciliation. In decisions that literally came down to the last instant, Congress enacted the legislation a few days before Christmas, 1982; President Reagan signed it into law in early January 1983.

Subcommittee Hearings on H.R. 5238

Hearings on the Orphan Drug Act introduced by Representative Waxman in December 1981 were held three months later, on March 8, 1982. The preliminary survey data, generated in the interim, were made public at the hearing. To Representative Waxman, the most notable fact in the survey was that during the previous decade, an average of only one marketed orphan drug per year had been sponsored and developed by pharmaceutical firms independent of government or university assistance. As he later noted during a press briefing, industry had marketed only about forty drugs for rare diseases, of which there were an estimated 2,000.[1]

Meanwhile, the PMA Commission on Drugs for Rare Diseases, whose formation had been announced almost exactly a year earlier, had been meeting once every two months since August 1981 and had defined its mission and scope by the time of these March 1982 hearings. Most of the commissioners were vice-presidents of major pharmaceutical firms. Two of the vice-presidents had been invited to testify at the hearings and had accepted, but neither was able to attend. Thus the impression was created, as one observer commented, that there were presidents and there were vice-presidents: The vice-presidents might be concerned about orphan drugs, but the presidents were in charge, were worried about the bottom line, and consequently were directing the vice-presidents to stay home. Industry's commitment to a solution was now in question. Were pharmaceutical company presidents not supporting legislation because they were relying on vice-presidents—namely, the PMA commission—to deal effectively with all problems? Or were there other reasons for the apparent boycott of the hearing? The answers were not forthcoming.

The PMA was represented by Peter Barton Hutt, a former FDA general counsel who had become an attorney with the Washington law firm of Covington and Burling. In his prepared statement, Hutt said industry was proud of its contributions toward developing nearly eighty drugs for rare diseases, but that the industry recognized the area deserved continued attention, as evidenced by its newly formed PMA Commission on Drugs for Rare Diseases. The PMA, said Hutt, supported the bill's approach of providing incentives to industry, but stressed the difficulties in defining an orphan drug strictly as one for a rare disease (citing, for instance, unpatentable drugs for common diseases, and rare-disease uses for marketed common-disease drugs). Instead, Hutt emphasized, the major problem was inflexibility of FDA's administrative policies on drug review. This problem applied to all drugs, not just those for rare diseases, he said, and suggested that rather than amending the Food, Drug and Cosmetic Act, Congress should await the outcome of FDA administrative changes recommended by various groups studying problems in the review process. For instance, he said, the PMA objected to the bill's provision that orphan drugs could be approved by FDA on the basis of one well-controlled study, as opposed to the conventional practice of relying on at least two studies. He argued that FDA already had that option—in fact, had used it recently to approve Timolol for preventing second heart attacks, based on only one (Norwegian) study—and suggested that FDA increase its use of this administrative option to speed the approval of drugs in general. His message was that the PMA did not feel the bill's regulatory or incentive provisions would solve the problem. Rather, streamlining FDA review processes in general would shorten review time and lessen development costs for all drugs, and this in turn would stimulate development of drugs for rare diseases.[2]

During questioning, Representative Waxman contradicted the industry's estimate of the number of industry-sponsored orphan drugs to date. He said PMA firms surveyed indicated that only fifty-eight drugs for rare diseases had been or were being developed, and that only ten marketed orphan drugs had been developed solely by industry. Waxman also pointed out that of the twenty-four industry-sponsored drugs in Compassionate IND status, sponsors of four said they did not intend to apply for an NDA, and only seven of the drugs currently had NDA applications under review by FDA. One drug had been in Compassionate IND status for nineteen years. Waxman asked Hutt if market incentives and regulatory provisions would not help place these drugs on the market.

Hutt responded that in some cases scientific problems were consigning the drugs to Compassionate IND status, but agreed that current FDA regulations do not distinguish between a Compassionate IND and an IND that is intended to go to the NDA stage. He concurred that this distinction should be made. Hutt emphasized, however, that there should not be a two-track system for drug approval—one for drugs for common diseases and another, expedited track for drugs for rare diseases. He stressed that streamlining FDA regulations for all drugs would, in the end, provide a greater incentive for companies to develop orphan drugs. Waxman, returning to the ten-drugs-in-ten-years figure, asked Hutt how the drug industry could state that it had and would continue to make significant contributions in the area of drugs for rare diseases and still assert that all that could be done had been done. Hutt countered that without industry participation, even in drugs primarily developed by government agencies, there would be no orphan drugs on the market today. Nevertheless, he said, industry would like to study the incentives provided in the legislation more closely, to see whether there were some provisions that could indeed by helpful.[3]

Assistant Secretary for Health Edward M. Brandt, Jr., testified that DHHS Secretary Richard Schweiker was that day announcing his intention to create a DHHS Orphan Products Board to coordinate federal activities on orphan products, including biologicals, medical devices, and diagnostic products as well as drugs. Brandt cited the government's already impressive record in developing orphan drugs by DHHS agencies, including twenty-six developed by NIH, thirty biologicals and drugs sponsored by CDC, and three drugs developed by institutes in ADAMHA. He stressed that any legislative changes made in the FFDCA law on behalf of orphan drugs should not change safety or efficacy requirements. He, like Hutt, emphasized there was no need for the bill's provision enabling orphan drugs to be approved on the basis of a single study, since FDA already had discretionary authority to do so. He also said FDA already permits Treatment INDs for using experimental drugs in patients when no therapeutic alternative exists, and that the Compassionate IND provision in the bill therefore was unnecessary. Finally, he said, economic incentives were important, but the Treasury Department opposed the tax credit provision in the bill. Both Assistant Secretary Brandt and FDA Commissioner Arthur Hull Hayes emphasized FDA's recently accelerated activities to coordinate FDA review and approval of orphan-drug applications, and to tailor requirements to fit existing pre-clinical testing limitations of certain orphan drugs.[4]

During questioning by Representative Waxman on how these federal activities would help drugs that were not profitable, the assistant secretary essentially proposed expanding the federal role in orphan drug development. He said the government would attempt to do a larger portion of the research required and would in many cases actually develop the drugs, as the NCI had been doing for some time.

Commissioner Hayes, asked to clarify the difference between Treatment INDs and Compassionate INDs, said there was no important difference. When asked how physicians learn the drugs are available, Hayes said information was disseminated primarily through drug references in published scientific literature, but added that the FDA would welcome any suggestions from the subcommittee on how to improve such efforts.

Finally, Marjorie Guthrie of the Committee to Combat Huntingtons Disease told subcommittee members they had heard from experts on the bill. Now she and others testifying as a panel were representing the people—the patients and their families who had waited for so long for help. Guthrie urged the members to recommend passage of legislation, even if imperfect; it would be a first step toward helping people with rare disorders who languish and die for want of a vigorous pursuit of treatment because none of the diseases afflicting them provides a market large enough to encourage major new drug efforts by the pharmaceutical industry.[5]

Redesigning the Legislation

Following the hearing, the fine tuning of the legislation took place. Assistant Secretary Brandt's announcement of the DHHS Board essentially preempted that provision in the Orphan Drug Act. Although the act's provision would stay in the bill to ensure its legal, as opposed to administrative, status, Representative Waxman and subcommittee staff were delighted; at a time when the Reagan administration was aggressively trying to cut down on government offices and functions, the department's announced intention to form a coordinating board came as a reassuring indication of progress.

A presentation on the orphan-drug situation, made shortly after the hearings during Ohio State University's annual seminar on pharmacy issues, caught the attention of Bill Haddad, president of the Generic Pharmaceutical Industry Association (GPIA). He was astounded, he said, to hear of the futile federal planning efforts and the fact that numbers of orphan drugs still were not sponsored, many presumably because of lack of patent protection. Haddad, who previously had considered orphan-drug problems to be beyond the province of the GPIA, became convinced otherwise and mobilized new GPIA efforts. The association provided strong support for the legislation and concurrently created the GPIA Orphan Drug Institute. Unlike the PMA commission, composed of industry vice-presidents, the GPIA institute was composed of chief executive officers (CEOs) of member firms, who could make both product and policy commitments on the spot. GPIA's break with the PMA position was a key factor in eventually securing general industry backing for the bill. The splitoff of one industry group to align itself with a bill's proponents is typical of the way compromises on controversial legislation eventually are reached: A major industry group (PMA) feels it must not stand alone in opposition to popularly-supported legislation and begins to worry that compromises reached with other industry groups will leave it without a hand in the important concessions reached.

After Haddad's move, PMA representatives lobbied for changes they wanted made in the bill. When compromises were forthcoming, so was their support for the legislation. The battle was far from over, however. The bill's supporters saw their hopes for enactment threatened, first by apparently irreconcilable differences between the House and the Senate on the issue of tax credits to industry, and next by rumors that the president would refuse to sign it into law because of Administration objections to a totally unrelated amendment attached as a rider to the bill. Final outcome of both controversies came down to the wire in a race against adjournment of the 97th Congress, when all legislation not enacted would automatically die.

The Bill Is Passed

Representative Waxman and the subcommittee's counsel, William Corr, spearheaded efforts to draft a final version of H.R. 5238, after intense discussion with industry, government, and academic research and consumer groups.

Two provisions in the draft that worried PMA were changed following discussions with subcommittee staff. First, industry was against postmarketing efficacy surveillance of orphan drugs following expedited FDA approval; this provision was deleted from the bill's final version. Second, PMA did not want a provision stipulating that FDA could approve an orphan candidate based on only one well-controlled study. Staff were sympathetic to PMA concerns that this provision implied more than one study was required for all other drugs, a misleading implication since FDA requirements on this point were not explicit. The PMA considered a far more important issue to be the lack of fit between FDA guidelines for orphan drugs and the requirements actually deemed necessary at the time of NDA review. This disparity, which had been emphasized in survey responses, added unnecessarily to development time and costs, according to the PMA, and was excess baggage unprofitable drugs did not need.

Thus the final House version of H.R. 5238 contained, instead, the provision that an orphan-drug sponsor may request written recommendations from FDA for nonclinical and clinical investigations that must be conducted before drug approval (or licensing, in the case of a biological product). FDA now would have to describe the number and type of animal and human clinical trials expected to be required for approval prior to the sponsors' initiation of studies. FDA practice had been to publish general guidelines for classes of drugs but not to respond to requests for guidance on specific drugs until human studies were underway. Staff anticipated that this new provision would be particularly helpful not only to industry but also to academic and federal agency scientists, who now would have some concept of the time and resources likely to be needed for drug approval before making any extensive resource commitments.

In the final House form, the bill, as described in the Committee Report, contained the following provisions, many of which had been retained from the bill as first introduced by Representative Waxman.[6] Based on the PMA-requested changes just described, Section 525 of Chapter V of the Food, Drug and Cosmetic Act was to be amended to require FDA to respond to requests from drug sponsors for written recommendations describing the number and type of animal and human clinical tests needed for approval. FDA's recommendation was to be based on the best information available at the time, and would not preclude revision if new scientific information became available before the drug was approved (or the biological was licensed). However, the committee expected such revisions only if the additional data were absolutely essential to assuring safety or efficacy. This replaced the bill's provision for FDA approval based on one well-controlled clinical trial.

Section 526 (unchanged) required FDA, upon a sponsor's request, to designate a drug as an orphan if the DHHS secretary defined it as a drug for a disease or condition occurring so infrequently in this country that there was no reasonable expectation that the development and distribution costs would be recovered from U.S. drug sales. The report explained that the term "rare in the United States" was used to assure that the bill's benefits applied to such drugs, even if those conditions or diseases for which they were intended were prevalent in other countries. It was further commented that if the bill encourages efforts on drugs needed in developing countries, that too was sound public policy. The section also required that public announcement be made of drugs designated as orphan, so that consumers and health professionals could become aware of their availability. This wavied the sponsor's right to trade secrecy about IND plans to test an experimental orphan drug.

Section 527 (unchanged) established a seven-year period of exclusive marketing for a sponsor from the date of FDA approval for an unpatentable orphan drug, based on the survey finding that a substantial number of orphan drugs were not eligible for a product patent.

Section 528 required FDA to encourage orphan-drug sponsors to design "open" protocols for human clinical tests. Their design should enable physicians treating patients not included in clinical trials to obtain the drug in the absence of alternative drug therapy. This provision was intended especially to improve access to those drugs being maintained indefinitely in Compassionate IND status. It was based on the survey finding that the average development time for such drugs was much longer than the norm, and that sponsors of some Compassionate IND drugs did not anticipate ever filing an NDA application for marketing the drug. Under the open protocol procedure, physicians could request the drug from the sponsor, who would have FDA's prior approval to add new individuals to the protocol. Both the drug sponsor and the requesting physician would have to collect any resulting clinical data requested by FDA.

The bill now no longer contained a section authorizing FDA to require manufacturers of approved orphan drugs to maintain an information collection system (post-marketing surveillance) on drug efficacy.

Section 3, amending Title II Section 227, of the Public Health Service Act, would establish the DHHS Orphan Products Board. The provision was preserved basically as originally introduced, but it was renamed Board instead of Committee, and its activities were expanded to include those for devices, in keeping with the board's initiatives begun prior to enactment of the legislation. The board was intended to promote development of orphan drugs and devices and to coordinate government activities. Additionally, it was to include in annual reports to Congress an evaluation of federal efforts to implement the act. The Committee on Energy and Commerce (the parent of the health subcommittee) deferred to the DHHS in not including members of the public or pharmaceutical companies on the board, but reported it planned to evaluate the board's performance and might later consider directing it to have broader participation.

Section 4, amending chapter 1 of the Internal Revenue Code of 1954 (relating to tax credits allowable) proposed a new Section 44H, "Clinical Testing Expenses for Certain Drugs for Rare Diseases or Conditions." The provision would allow a tax credit for any pharmaceutical company developing an orphan drug, in an amount equal to 50 percent of costs of conducting human clinical tests in any taxable year. The remaining 50 percent of costs could be considered a deductible business expense, providing a total tax liability reduction of 73 percent of the clinical testing costs of an orphan drug. The bill limited the tax credit to those clinical trials specifically involving orphan indications, since drugs may undergo simultaneous trials for orphan and nonorphan indications. Certain limitations of this provision have been criticized by pharmaceutical sponsors (discussed later). The tax credit would be available through December 31, 1989, and would be monitored carefully by the committee, informed in part by specifics to be provided by the Orphan Products Board on federal revenue loss associated with the provision.

Total costs in carrying out H.R. 5238 were estimated to be $9 million in the first year following enactment and in 1990, and $18 million annually in each of the interim fiscal years, according to a Congressional Budget Office estimate contained in the report. The six provisions (plus a seventh added by the Senate, discussed next) are summarized in Table 7–1.

While the bill was being readied for House passage, a conference on orphan drugs was held on September 27 and 28, 1982, sponsored by the University of Michigan, and organized by two orphan-drug researchers there, George Brewer and Jess Thoene. During the two-day conference, representatives from several of the voluntary health organizations met to discuss how to most effectively work for passage of the legislation. Up to that time, they had mounted separate lobbying efforts. Historically, in fact, they had competed for the attention of Congress and the NIH, each voluntary agency seeking increased funding for research on a specific disease.

For instance, Marjorie Guthrie had been particularly effective in

Table 7–1
Provisions of P.L. 97-414

1. FDA is to provide recommendations for investigations of drugs intended for use in rare diseases or conditions on request.
2. FDA is to designate drugs for rare diseases or conditions, on request, if the secretary finds that to be the case, based on facts and circumstances available at the date the designation is made.
3. A seven-year period of market exclusivity is provided for unpatentable drugs, beginning on the date the drug is approved by FDA.
4. FDA is required to encourage sponsors to design open protocols for drug availability to patients not included in clinical trials.
5. DHHS is authorized to create an Orphan Products Board to coordinate and evaluate federal orphan-drug and device activities.
6. Tax credits of 50 percent are provided in any taxable year of the costs of human clinical trials for orphan indications. The remaining 50 percent of such costs are deductible, resulting in a total reduction in tax liability of 73 percent of the costs of such trials.
7. The DHHS secretary is authorized to make grants and enter into contracts for orphan-drug clinical trials; authorizations are $4 million each for FY 1983, FY 1984, and FY 1985.

lobbying for Huntingtons disease and had played a major role in convincing congress to establish the Commission on Huntingtons Disease and its Consequences, on which she served as chairperson. She soon became convinced from the commission's deliberations and studies that not only were problems faced by Huntingtons patients and their families similar to those encountered by all patients with rare debilitating conditions, but that research targeted to a particular disease was not likely to produce results any faster than broad support for basic research in general.

Guthrie had become a strong advocate of a united approach by voluntary agencies. Although she was not at the Michigan Orphan Drug meeting—she had developed a type of cancer that could not be arrested or cured—members of voluntary agencies had heard her appeals for a cooperative approach and at the Michigan meeting joined together to form the National Organization for Rare Disorders (NORD). Together, they would push for congressional passage of the Orphan Drug bill, which had been rumored to have powerful opponents in the Senate because of the tax credit provisions. Such temporary alliances of groups that are often in competition or even opposition is essential to enactment of almost any controversial legislation. In this case, however, NORD members were planning to maintain a lasting alliance to work together on problems posed by rare diseases. The Orphan Drug bill was passed by the House—

literally, just as NORD formed at this first meeting on September 28, 1984.

The fate of the legislation in the Senate was in doubt. The bill, introduced by Senator Nancy Kassebaum, had not been reported out of the Labor and Human Resources Committee, chaired by Senator Orrin Hatch (R-Utah). In what became a feedback loop, however, art now imitated life in a new "Quincy" episode. Actor Jack Klugman and his television crew had been kept apprised of the tortuous path of the legislation since his congressional appearance in support of an orphan-drug bill. After Klugman and company heard in early August 1982 that even if the Waxman bill passed the House, it was likely to die in the Senate because several key senators opposed the tax credit provision, their cameras started rolling again. In the new episode, which aired at about the time the bill was being considered by the House, Senate consideration was dramatized as being held up by one senator's objections to extending tax credits to industry. About 500 patients with rare diseases who had been contacted through the voluntary agency network were filmed marching toward the Capitol in hopes of freeing the first bill that might someday free them. At the end of the episode, in a line which in real life had been used by another federal official involved in the legislation, the senator said he could not support the measure but would not try to block it. The "Quincy" show revived the public consciousness of orphan drugs. But this time it came while congressional negotiations were in progress, adding heat to an already intense situation.

After H.R. 5238 passed the House, Representative Waxman was anxious for Senate action on the bill in some form before the Congress recessed for a short break and then returned for the so-called lame-duck session after the November election. During the lame-duck session, Congress was committed to acting only on measures that already were near final passage. Therefore, if any version of an Orphan Drug bill passed the Senate before the recess, there was the possibility that difference between the House and Senate versions could be worked out through negotiation before members returned. The final measure then could be passed by both Houses.

In this atmosphere, Representative Waxman met with senators Hatch and Edward Kennedy (D-Mass.) and others to urge them to push a bill through the Senate before the recess. Achieving consensus of key senators, according to Susan Hattan of Senator Kassebaum's office, required nothing short of a marathon of meetings, which literally came right down to the recess bell. During a meeting that ran from 10 P.M. September 30 until 10 A.M. the following morning (recess day), staff from the offices of senators Hatch,

Kennedy, Kassebaum, Robert Dole (R-Kan., chairman of Senate Finance Committee, which had jurisdiction over the tax credit provision in the bill), and Russell B. Long (D-La., ranking member of that committee) met to work out a version of the Waxman bill that might be acceptable to them all. This group decided to drop the tax credit from the bill because both senators Dole and Long were adamantly against the provision. Moreover, it settled the question of whether Senator Hatch's Labor and Human Resources Committee or Senator Dole's Finance Committee would have jurisdiction over the bill: Without the tax credit provision the Finance Committee could not claim jurisdiction. In place of a tax credit, under Section 5 of the bill, a provision was added authorizing the DHHS secretary to spend $4 million in each of the fiscal years 1983, 1984, and 1985 for grants for drugs for rare diseases, and to enter into contracts for human clinical trials necessary for the development of orphan drugs. With this major controversy resolved, the Senate's bill soon became a legislative Christmas tree on which was hung seven additional amendments, most of them on health care but none of them directly related to orphan drugs. By unanimous consent, the Senate, on this last day of the pre-recess period, discharged the Labor and Human Resources Committee from further consideration of the bill it had listed on its calendar. In the same motion the Senate took up the redrafted version and passed it within hours of the recess bell.

In the interim before Congress returned for the post-election lame-duck session, negotiations took place between House and Senate staff on differences between the House and Senate-passed bills. House aides also met with staff of the Senate Finance Committee to urge reinstitution of the tax credit. According to one account, Senator Dole had relaxed his opposition to this measure after a lobbying visit from Sharon Dobkin, the young New York woman with myoclonus. During the visit, Senate bells rang, announcing an imminent roll call vote. The sudden sound of the bells triggered her myoclonus, causing her to jerk uncontrollably. Reportedly, thereafter Senator Dole had been swayed to consider a tightened tax credit provision. Finally, according to Susan Hattan, during a meeting with representatives from the Treasury Department, the Joint House-Senate Tax Committee, the Senate Finance Committee, the House Subcommittee on Health and the Environment, and staff from senators Kassebaum's and Hatch's offices, new language for the tax credit provision was hammered out. The result was a tightened provision— one that participants agreed held little room for abuse or massive drains on Treasury funds.

Thereafter, the further amended version of H.R. 5238, which now contained both the tax credit and the $4 million grants authorization, and seven other amendments unrelated to the act, was passed by the House on December 14 and by the Senate three days later. One of its amendments, however, carried the potential for precipitating a presidential pocket veto, which would occur if President Reagan failed to sign the bill by January 4, the last day of the period stipulated by law and too late for the then-adjourned 97th Congress to overturn a veto. The suspense arose from one of the amendments to the Orphan Drug bill sponsored by Utah's Senator Hatch. It called for a federal investigation of the possibility that nuclear testing in Nevada had caused thyroid cancer in citizens of the neighboring state of Utah.

This amendment instructed the DHHS secretary to conduct research necessary to: develop valid and credible assessments of the risks of thyroid cancer associated with doses of iodine-131; estimate thyroid doses of iodine-131 received by individuals from nuclear bomb fallout; and estimate those doses received by people in the state neighboring the Nevada atmospheric nuclear bomb tests. The secretary was to publish radioepidemiological tables estimating the probability of specific radiation doses causing human cancers. The tables were to be accompanied by evaluations of their credibility, validity, and degree of certainty, and a compilation of formulas on which the probabilities were based; tables were to be updated every four years or whenever deemed necessary by the secretary.[7]

Rumors of the president's reluctance to sign the bill were mounting. Adverse reports from the Office of Management and Budget and the departments of the Treasury and Justice, which were opposed both to the tax credits and the Utah testing amendment, signaled to many proponents that a pocket veto was likely. But although these concerns contributed to the president's reported inclination to allow the bill to die, there was still some optimism that he might sign, based on the premise that the Orphan Drug Act was in keeping with the Reagan administration's philosophy of enhancing private-sector initiatives as opposed to increasing the federal role in orphan-drug development as Assistant Secretary Brandt had indicated might happen. Additionally, since it seemed to be a bill with widespread public appeal, supporters decided to harness this public sentiment.

First, a press conference was organized by Abbey Meyers, the federal affairs liaison of NORD (the newly established coalition of voluntary health agencies). The press conference was called to focus public attention directly on congressional passage of the Orphan Drug bill and, indirectly, to pursuade the president to sign it into law. The conference was far from glamorous, recalled Meyers, who had been a moving force among voluntary agency members in supporting the legislation. As a mother of three children with Tourette syndrome, she had testified at the hearings and had helped organize NORD. Meyers recalled that reporters, assembled in a Capitol hearing room, told the speakers—including Sharon Dobkin, Representative Waxman, Senator Hatch, Lewis Engman of the PMA, and Bill Haddad of the GPIA—to make it quick because the media had another press conference to cover in fifteen mintues.[8] Representative Waxman told reporters that Congress regarded the bill as an essential part of a national commitment to develop more drugs for rare diseases, and said he hoped the president would realize that too. Bill Haddad said the orphan-drug bill was the "golden egg of the lame duck Congress."

Still, there was no indication the president would sign. As the pocket veto date neared, House subcommittee staff called newspaper editors around the country urging editorial support for Waxman's orphan-drug bill. They met with overwhelming success. With one day left, NORD placed full-page ads in the *Washington Post* and the *L.A. Times* imploring the president to sign a bill of hope for patients with rare diseases and conditions, and urging people to call the White House in support. NORD estimates 50,000 people did just that. Among them, according to one source, were a number of actresses favoring the law who were enlisted to add their persuasion to the effort through calls to Mrs. Reagan. The next day, January 4, 1983, President Reagan signed P.L. 97–414 into law.

Democratic Representative Waxman commended his Republican congressional colleagues, Representative Edward Madigan (R-Ill., ranking minority member of his subcommittee) and Senator Hatch, for their efforts to explain the legislation to the White House. He commended the voluntary health organization members for their diligence in support of the legislation. Finally, he commended the president for recognizing its importance and signing it into law.[9] An announcement of the president's action sealing the new law would make the evening news telecasts.

Bill Corr called Abbey Meyers that day to tell her the president was going to sign the bill. Then a reporter called her for comment, saying he was live (on the air); Meyers, usually loquacious, said she was speechless for the first time in a long while: It felt, she told him, as though she were giving birth after three years in labor. One orphan-drug clinical researcher, who had been active in the crusade for the legislation, sent her a dozen roses. Someone from the Tourette Syndrome Association presented her with a bottle of champagne. When she went home, roses and champagne in hand, her children asked where supper was; it was late and they were hungry. So, she said, the victory never had a chance to go to her head. But there was new reason for hope. Bill Corr, who had spent much of the afternoon calling major supporters of the bill to announce the president's decision to sign, packed his briefcase with the night's work on one of the subcommittee's pending issues, and headed home.

Notes

1. D'Vera Cohn, "Orphan Drugs," United Press International, December 21, 1982.

2. Peter Barton Hutt, "Statement," *Orphan Drug Hearing*, March 8, 1982, (Washington, D.C.: U.S. Government Printing Office, 1982), Serial No. 97-128, pp. 283–299.

3. Edward M. Brandt, Jr., "Statement," Ibid., pp. 316–320, 329–340.

4. Arthur Hull Hayes, "Statement," Ibid., pp. 316–320, 329–340.

5. Marjorie Guthrie, "Statement," Ibid., pp. 299–301.

6. Orphan Drug Act Report, 97th Congress, 2nd Session, House Rept. 97-840, Part 1, September 17, 1982.

7. Congressional Record, October 1, 1982, pp. S13219–S13227.

8. Abbey Meyers, personal communication, April 9, 1984.

9. Representative Henry A. Waxman, press release, January 4, 1983.

8
New Plans, New Planners, New Problems, and New Vistas

Befefore orphan drugs became an idea in good currency, NIH officials had emphasized during appropriations hearings that a large number of Americans (constituents) are afflicted with various diseases and conditions requiring increased research efforts to develop effective treatment or prevention. Now rare diseases were legitimate, too. In the neurological field alone there are about 600 rare diseases. As Murray Goldstein, director of the National Institute of Neurological and Communicative Disorders and Stroke (NINCDS) quipped, he now could introduce himself as head of the orphan disease institute; it was a lot easier to say.

During the interval between introduction of orphan-drug legislation and its eventual enactment into law, industry and government established formal means to facilitate development and availability of known orphan drugs. This time, the efforts of one were not entirely independent of those of the other. Evaluation of the effectiveness and efficiency of these new measures is still some time off, but perhaps an account of early returns may suggest some trends worth watching.

In analyzing orphan-drug actions by the private and public sectors, it is useful to evaluate the results to date, and also the underlying planning processes and policy decisions. A chronological listing of some of the major events, provided in Table 8–1, gives an indication of the temporal relationship between public- and private-sector actions, including those by voluntary agencies.

The Beginning of Interactive Planning

The PMA Commission on Drugs for Rare Diseases, which began meeting on a bimonthly basis in August 1981, has served a vital function as a central clearinghouse for information on known orphan drugs. Moreover, it has begun to broaden its original, narrowly defined, mission. In so doing, it has the potential for becoming what

Table 8–1

Chronology of Some Major Initiatives, Public and Private Sectors

1. March 1981—PMA Commission on Drugs for Rare Diseases announced; first meeting, August 11, 1981.
2. March 1981—Congressman Whitten's appropriation for FDA Office of Orphan Products Development; Office established in May 1982.
3. March 1982—DHHS Orphan Products Board announced.
4. April 1982—GPIA Orphan Drug Institute formed.
5. September 28, 1982—Orphan Drug bill passed by the U.S. House of Representatives; Orphan Drugs and Diseases Conference held, University of Michigan; National Organization for Rare Diseases (NORD) formed.
6. December 14, 1982—Amended Orphan Drug bill (H.R. 5238) passed the House; bill passed the Senate on December 17, 1982.
7. January 4, 1983—President Reagan signed H.R. 5238, completing enactment of Public Law (P.L.) 97-414.
8. May 1983—Symposium on Orphan Products, organized by FDA, sponsored by Sandoz.
9. September and November 1983—FDA Orphan Products Development Office announced its first grant awards.
10. January 30, 1984—Second request for proposals for grants funded under the Whitten orphan-drug appropriation.
11. March 1984—Orphan Drugs Symposium, held at Mount Sinai Hospital and Medical Center, sponsored by PMA, GPIA, FDA, and Myoclonus Research Fund.
12. June 24, 1984—Introduction of the Drug Price Competition and Patent Term Restoration Act of 1984 (H.R. 3605) by Representative Waxman providing market exclusivity for unpatentable drugs as part of a generic drug bill.

Eric Trist, a systems research pioneer, would call a "referent organization."[1] This is a key organization which acts as a central focus or referent through which other groups or organizations interact, either formally or informally, both with it and with one another.

PMA commission chairman is Theodore Cooper, an executive vice-president of the Upjohn Company. Now an industry leader, he also has been a major official of the NIH, an assistant secretary for health under the Ford administration, and dean of the Cornell Medical School. Cooper, who has seen the problems of orphan drugs from several vantage points, is a boundary spanner who has an excellent opportunity to bring different perspectives to the attention of the commission and, from there, to other companies and groups involved in orphan-drug planning. Several other commission members have spoken out in the past on problems of orphan drugs; they include Lewis Sarett of Merck, Barry Bloom of Pfizer, and Pedro Cuatrecases of Burroughs Wellcome. Several have worked closely with academia.

Functioning in its clearinghouse role, the PMA commission has encouraged developers of drugs for rare diseases to provide information on the drug's scientific potential, to be evaluated by commissioners and outside consultants. Favorably reviewed applications are circulated to member companies to stimulate additional research or commercial development.

Although the main focus is on drugs or devices for use in rare diseases or conditions in the United States, the commission has not excluded review of candidates for diseases which are rare in this country but endemic to other nations. As described in the commission's 1982 Annual Report, priority for review occurs in this order: (1) proposals for drugs with safety and efficacy data considered adequate by the investigator or commission for NDA submission; (2) proposals involving INDs with demonstrated safety and/or efficacy established in phase I, II, or III clinical studies; (3) research leads involving a new chemical entity with preclinical or other scientific evidence of efficacy and no absolute contraindications; and (4) proposals concerning new uses, formulations, or combinations of marketed products, which are referred to the drug's current commercial sponsor for their possible submission of a supplemental NDA. The report emphasizes that ordinarily none of the submitted information is considered confidential. If proprietary data are critical to the review, they are accepted, provided the submitter has taken the necessary legal measures to protect them.[2] This policy ensued after some commission members expressed concern that sponsors of orphan drugs should not have proprietary rights jeopardized by this review process.

Early in the commission's life, FDA's J. Richard Crout wrote to his long-time associate Theodore Cooper suggesting that an FDA liaison be invited to participate. His was a key step toward positioning the commission to take a lead in coordinating federal and industry orphan-drug plans. Shortly thereafter liaison invitations were extended to CDC and NIH. Additionally, members of voluntary health organizations and academic researchers have attended meetings on an intermittent—in some cases regular—basis.

William Corr discussed the planned Waxman orphan-drug survey with the commissioners at the December 1981 meeting, and he and Susan Hatten of Senator Kassebaum's office have followed the group's progress at several meetings. FDA liaisons Marion Finkel and Stuart Nightingale have presented descriptions of Orphan Product Development Office activities, provided clarification of the treatment IND program, and sought PMA commission assistance in locating sponsors for several orphan-drug cases coming to FDA's attention. This marks the first systematic PMA-FDA cooperation on specific drugs.

Saul Schepartz of NCI and Murray Goldstein of NINCDS, as NIH liaison, have described various NIH drug R&D programs and the many mechanisms, past and present, used to collaborate with industry. Additionally, Goldstein provided results of a survey he conducted to define the number and nature of NIH drug projects and industry relationships. He found that of the twelve institutes surveyed, formal programs of drug development and evaluation were underway intramurally (in NIH laboratories) in three institutes, through grants in four institutes, and through contracts in five institutes. Additionally, five institutes had grants pertaining to rare-disease drugs, which were not part of a formal program. Formal and informal activities included performing chemical characterization, animal toxicity, and clinical testing for phases I, II, and III, with a slight predilection for formal arrangements for biochemical collaboration and informal arrangements in clinical testing. Finally, the survey indicated that officials of seven institutes wished to explore additional R&D arrangements with industry.

Commission members have heard from CDC officials of that agency's need for increased industry participation in several biologicals it has developed or distributes. The most pressing problem, according to Lynn Shans of CDC, has been to locate a commercial source of pentamidine to treat AIDS patients with pneumocystis carinii pneumonia. At the time, CDC's supplies were perilously depleted and soon would be insufficient to meet the AIDS need. It was the GPIA, not the PMA, however, that intervened in this situation. GPIA president William Haddad and Kenneth Larsen of GPIA member company Zenith went to Europe and negotiated with May & Baker, Ltd. in England to continue to provide the drug, which the British company previously had sold only in small quantities and was about to discontinue. May & Baker, Ltd. supplies are expected to be ample until domestic production by PMA member LyphoMed are developed and approved by FDA.[3]

Initially, the PMA commission was busy with applications of known orphan drugs whose developers had not yet found commercial sponsors. The commission received twenty-three inquiries in 1982 and sixteen inquiries in the first half of 1983. Thereafter (as of February 1984), inquiries dwindled to three. The disposition of these inquiries and reviews is contained in Tables 8–2, 8–3, and 8–4. As Cooper put it, the commission suddenly was underwhelmed. This situation was not unanticipated, however. Representative Waxman and others had predicted that early federal and private efforts would center on a backlog of known drug candidates in need of commercial sponsors. Thereafter, efforts would be far less visible, such as stimulating the use of incentives contained in the new law, and finding commercial sponsors for new drugs which may become developed by academic scientists if they are convinced that such drugs can be

Table 8–2
PMA Commission: Disposition of Formal Proposals Approved[a]

Drug	Condition	Sponsor
1-5HTP	Post-anoxic myoclonus	Bolar Pharmaceutical[b]
Trien	Wilsons Disease	Merck & Co., Inc.
Hematin	Acute porphyria	Abbott Laboratories
I[131] Inodonorcholesterol	Adrenal gland tumor diagnosis	Mallinckrodt, Inc.
Phosphocysteamine	Nephropathic cystinosis	Grant made by PMA member firms
Antiglucocorticoids	Cushings Disease	Roussel-UCLAF
Oxymetholone (5 mg. tablets)	Hereditary angioedema	Syntex (USA)
Iridium 191	Detecting shunts in cardiac septal defects	Being solicited
Zinc Acetate	Wilsons disease	Being solicited
Dithiocarb	Nickel poisoning	Awaiting FDA requirements before soliciting sponsor

[a]Adapted from "PMA Commission Inquiries and Proposals Received through February 1, 1984," provided at April 1984 meeting.
[b]GPIA firm.

systematically transformed into sponsored products. At this juncture, the PMA commission is exploring the nature of its future role. Among those suggested by Cooper at the July 1984 PMA Commission meeting is a study of drug pathology and toxicology "bottlenecks" impeding drug development by academic researchers, and support of other studies, workshops and symposia. Commission vice-chairman George Goldstein also recommended sponsoring information activities on orphan drug development for academic scientists.

Concurrently—somewhat less visibly but no less effectively—the GPIA, with its Institute for Orphan Drugs, is forging into several new areas as the generic industry's referent organization for orphan drugs. Its method to date, as illustrated earlier in the pentamidine example, has been largely crisis intervention. When quick, decisive action is required, the GPIA can respond because, as described earlier, the GPIA institute is composed of company CEOs. Commitments can be made at meetings where the problems are first introduced. This was the case in providing emergency funding for Jesse Thoene's studies on phosphocysteamine for treating the kidney-destroying illness cystinosis. Thoene's original study of this fatal metabolic disease in children had involved cysteamine, which proved to have too objectionable a taste and odor (Thoene's difficulties with trade secret

Table 8–3
PMA Commission: Disposition of Other Formal Proposals Received

Drug	Condition
Review pending	
Methylated mitotane	Adrenolytic agent
Sn-protoporphyrin	Neonatal jaundice
Alpha keto analogues (citrulline and arginine)	Ureagenesis defects
Proposals rejected	
U series	Downs syndrome
Syncardon (device)	Arteriolar occlusive disease
Referred to DHHS	
Alpha galactosidase	Fabrys disease
Diaspirins	Sickle cell anemia
Pseudomonas vaccine	Cell-free preparation needed
3 basic research studies	
Revision requested	
Tetrahydrobiopterin	Phenylketonuria
Referred to original manufacturer for special packaging, formulation	
Combination product	Leprosy

Source: Adapted from "PMA Commission Inquiries and Proposals Received Through February 1, 1984," provided at April 1984 PMA meeting.

Table 8–4
PMA Commission: Disposition of Inquiries Received[a]

Total Received	17
Pending	2
Rejected	2
Formal proposal requested	10
Outside commission's scope	3[b]

Source: Adapted from "PMA Commission Inquiries and Proposals Received Through February 1, 1984," presented at April 1984 PMA commission meeting.

[a]Formal and informal.

[b]Includes inquiries concerning: new uses for marketed drugs, referred to original NDA holder; reimbursement for investigational drugs by third-party payers, referred to DHHS; and financial support of basic research.

status of cysteamine were described in chapter 4). With the change to phosphocysteamine, however, FDA had required new safety data, and Thoene had exhausted his limited funds in trying to supply this data. To keep his studies alive and to ensure continuity, the GPIA extended some emergency funding to the University of Michigan researcher. A GPIA member company is sponsoring Theone's current work, along with grants from both the PMA and the FDA. GPIA-member firm Bolar Pharmaceutical has become the sponsor of l-5HTP for use in postanoxic myoclonus, ending Melvin Van Woert's nearly decade-long search for a commercial sponsor. The GPIA Institute also helped to forge a new collaborative effort between two GPIA member firms (Henry Schein Inc. and Rugby Laboratories) and PMA member Sandoz to fund development of zinc therapy for Wilson's disease by George Brewer at the University of Michigan.

Among its more long-term efforts, the GPIA has helped to organize and provide startup monies for a recently established fundraising organization, the National Orphan Drugs and Devices Foundation, headed by Joel Bennett. In collaboration with NORD (National Organization for Rare Disorders), GPIA is developing a computerized information clearinghouse on orphan diseases, including names of researchers, available therapies (if any), and names of voluntary organizations. The on-line service will be available to practicing physicians and, at the start, will include information on about thirty to forty diseases identified by NORD. The GPIA plans to coordinate this service with any federal efforts that may emerge from current discussions within the DHHS board. In response to an article on the computerized service in the Institute's magazine *Generics*, about 200 physicians have written requesting additional information on its use.[4]

Finally, the institute helped stimulate a new orphan-drug distribution effort by major drug chains, including Revco, Rugby Laboratories Inc. and Henry Schein Inc., providing marketed orphan drugs on request to participating pharmacists at essentially no net profit.[5] According to Patrick Donoho of Revco, the program is intended to ensure that patients have rapid access to orphan products prescribed, since pharmacists rarely stock products that are infrequently requested. Additionally, Revco expects to raise pharmacist and physician awareness about the existence of orphan products. Since drugs are provided at no net profit to the wholesaler or Revco retailers, Donoho says, this should stimulate competition among retailers, which ultimately could benefit patients in terms of lower orphan-drug prices. His conjecture may be supported by results of the orphan-drug survey that suggested that high distribution costs are associated with higher than average retail costs to the consumer. This direct distribution program may help ease that problem. Finally, Revco helped strengthen voluntary agency efforts by providing $8,000 in startup funding to NORD.[6]

The FDA Office of Orphan Products Development

Meanwhile, the FDA Office of Orphan Products Development, established by the Whitten amendment to FDA's appropriations bill in 1982, continued efforts begun in the late 1970s to expedite approval of products for rare diseases and to seek commercial sponsors. Stuart Nightingale, associate commissioner for health affairs, outlined FDA orphan-drug activities in these general areas: (1) identifying and monitoring adequacy of available data by reviewing all investigator-sponsored INDs semiannually; (2) reviewing literature reports of marketed drugs being used, though unapproved, for orphan diseases; (3) assisting in preparing orphan-drug protocols and compiling data; (4) specifying studies needed for FDA approval; (5) tailoring approval requirements for orphan drugs; (6) using Public Health Service laboratories when necessary for drugs with high priority or promise; (7) providing technical assistance in preparing NDAs; and (8) conducting priority review of orphan-drug applications.[7]

Even before enactment of P.L. 97-414, therefore, FDA had announced its intentions to expedite review procedures for orphan drugs, or, as Nightingale referred to it, to systematize and focus previous ad hoc efforts on behalf of the products. FDA already had approved fourteen such products between 1978 and 1981 (Table 8–5). Because these drugs were approved before enactment of the Orphan Drug Act, however, sponsors are not eligible for the act's benefits.

In 1983, FDA awarded twelve orphan product development grants totaling $500,000 from FDA's appropriations amendment (Table 8–6). Grant applications are reviewed in much the same way that NIH grants are reviewed—by an advisory council, which makes funding recommendations. The final decision on FDA grants lies with the director of the FDA Office of Orphan Products Development.

Also in 1983 the FDA approved six orphan products (Table 8–7), only one of which (hematin) is officially designated as an orphan and therefore eligible for incentives under the act. The con-

Table 8–5
Orphan Drugs Approved by FDA between 1978 and 1981[a]

Drug	Condition
Drugs in which FDA or NIH assisted	
Vidarabine[c]	Viral encephalitis
Natamycin[b,c]	Rare fungal infections
Metyrosine[b,c]	Pheochromocytoma
Isosulfan Blue[b,d]	Lymph node visualization
Potassium Iodide[b,d]	Thyroid block in radiation emergency
Aminoglutethamide[b]	Adrenal function suppression in Cushings disease
Other orphan drugs approved	
Dantrolene sodium	Malignant hyperthermia
Calcitriol	Hypocalcemia in dialysis patients
Desmopressin	Antidiuretic
Metoclopropamide	Muscle stimulant for gastroparesis
Alprostadil (PGE$_1$)	Presurgical treatment for infant congenital heart defects
Bretylium Tosylate	Ventricular arrhythmias
Calcifediol	Low blood calcium treatment
Saralasin Acetate	Hypertension detection

Source: Adapted from *Orphan Drugs Approved between 1978 and 1981*, FDA.

[a]Approved before the orphan-drug law and not eligible for provisions under the law.

[b]FDA solicited NDA submission or sought manufacturer.

[c]NIH funded or conducted studies.

[d]FDA assembled data or conducted laboratory studies.

fusion stems from the dual origin of FDA orphan-drug authorizations. Under the Whitten FDA appropriation amendment, products considered to be for rare diseases or conditions are to receive special handling (primarily expedited review and assistance) by the newly established FDA Office for Orphan Products Development. The office includes under this heading not only drugs for rare diseases, but also devices, veterinary products, and medical foods. The Orphan Drug Act of 1983 applies to drugs and biologicals only, and provides the tax and market exclusivity incentives. Only drugs whose sponsors specifically request and are granted an orphan designation, under FDA guidelines to be described later, are eligible for the incentives provided by the Act.

After the P.L. 97-414 was signed into law, FDA officials drafted implementation guidelines. Many specifics still await approval by

Table 8–6
Orphan-Product Grant Awards by FDA, September and November 1983

Grantee[a]	$ in 1000s[b]	Drug	Condition
Rockefeller University	$112.1	Phenytoin	Epidermolysis bullosa
Rockefeller University	$60.6	WR 2721	Cystinuria
University of Michigan	$66.9	Pantethine	Nephropathic cystinosis
University of Michigan	$45.2	131 I-MIGB	Pheochromocytoma
Adria Laboratories Inc.	$50.4	Mesna	Cyclophosphamide-induced cystitis prevention
NYS Psychiatric Institute	$92.0	Imipramine	Prepubertal depression
University of California (L.A.)	$50.4	Fenfluramine	Autism
Mount Sinai School of Medicine	$22.3	Harmaline	Cerebellar disorders
University of Iowa	$80.0	Chlorambucil	Progressive systemic sclerosis
Childrens Hospital & Research Foundation (Oh.)	$50.6	VIL	Phenylketonuria
Case Western Reserve	$44.8	Carbonyl Iron	Iron deficiency anemia
JFK Institute	$54.5	DMPS	Child lead poisoning

Source: Adapted from "Grant Awards, Office of Orphan Products Development, FDA, September and November 1983," available from FDA.

[a]Grants awarded to individual investigators at these institutions.

[b]First year funding amounts.

other federal agencies and departments, such as the Internal Revenue Service (IRS), the Office of Management and Budget (OMB), and the Justice Department. Industry has been making its case and awaiting the outcome.

Interim guidelines for implementing Section 526, designating drugs as orphans, initially set U.S. prevalence (the number of people with the disease or condition at any one time), at 100,000. As a result of public comments (routinely invited in response to proposed guidelines and regulations issued by government agencies), especially by voluntary health organizations, the maximum figure for eligibility was raised to 200,000 to cover drugs and biologicals for orphan diseases whose prevalence was on the large side of a small market. The 200,000 figure may apply to subsets (subpopulations) of those with

Table 8–7
Orphan Products Approved by FDA in 1983[a]

Drug	Sponsor
Sodium cellulose phosphate (Calcibind)	Mission Pharmacal
Acetohydroxamic acid (Lithostat)	Mission Pharmacal
Hematin[b] (Panhematin)	Abbott
Alpha fetoprotein (AFP) diagnostic kit[c]	Abbott
Chenodiol (Chenix)	Rowell
Etoposide (VePesid)	Bristol Myers

Source: Adapted in part from *Scrip,* January 30, 1984, No. 866, p. 11, and from Roger Gregorio, FDA, personal communication, June 1984.

[a]All but one of these drugs lack an official orphan designation by FDA under guidelines implementing the Orphan Drug Act, and therefore are not currently eligible for incentives under the law. Trade names are in parentheses.

[b]Drug has been designated orphan under the Act.

[c]A device.

more common diseases or conditions, if the drug is to be labeled exclusively for that subgroup. For vaccines or other prophylactics, the prevalence figure applies to the number of vaccinations per year. Sponsors of diagnostic drugs used for 200,000 or fewer people per year, however, must supply additional information (to be described) to obtain an orphan designation.

Under the guidelines, the sponsor is to provide: (1) a statement requesting an orphan designation; (2) a description of the disease or condition for which the product will be investigated; and (3) a statement of understanding that the sponsor's name, the generic and trade name of the drug, and the proposed indication will be made public. Additionally, the sponsor is to provide an estimate of the size and demographics of the intended U.S. patient population, and the rationale for the drug's use, including a brief summary of the pharmacologic or clinical data supporting it.

For drugs intended for more than 200,000 people in this country (or for diagnostic drugs intended for 200,000 or fewer people per year) additional information in support of an orphan designation is required. These data should demonstrate, in keeping with the law, that the disease or condition occurs so infrequently in the United States that there is no reasonable expectation of recovering costs from U.S. sales. The required information includes: (1) estimated costs for developing and distributing the drug, and (2) estimated U.S. sales on which the sponsor has concluded those costs will not be recovered, either during the drug's remaining patent life or—in the case of unpatentable drugs—during the seven-year exclusive marketing of the drug. Anticipated costs related to the Orphan Drug Act include those for collecting data and holding meetings in support of gaining an orphan designation, determining drug patentability, screening and conducting animal and clinical studies, preparing the IND and NDA or product license application, possibly distributing the drug under a Treatment IND, developing a dosage form; distributing and promoting the drug, keeping records and reports, licensing a drug obtained from another source, obtaining liability insurance, and paying costs of depreciation and overhead related to the orphan drug.

Anticipated U.S. sales should be based on a reasonable projection of future revenues, considering intended market size, the drug's degree of safety and efficacy, availability of other agents and therapies (including any likelihood that superior agents will become available), and estimated postmarket patent life or market exclusivity.

Guidelines stipulate that FDA will inform the sponsor of its decision within sixty days after receipt of the designation request. As of June 1984, FDA had received more than twenty drug designation applications, of which sixteen were granted (Table 8–8). FDA officials have been surprised at the relative lack of applications to date. The implications are not clear, but the situation could reflect industry's intention to await determination of tax and patent guidelines. Other possible factors include a lack of suitable candidates; reluctance to provide cost and revenue estimates; or disappointment over the extent of incentives. Of the more than nine sponsors whose drugs were not designated as orphan, some were unable to show an estimated loss, while others eschewed the paperwork involved in applying for the designation. Sponsors can request orphan designation for drugs that already are under development, as well as for new INDs. Provisions will be retroactive to January 4, 1983, when the law was signed. Unpatentable drugs approved one year prior to the law can be designated as orphan after the fact and receive the seven-year market exclusivity protection.

Reportedly the FDA has identified 300 potential orphan-drug candidates from among INDs filed with FDA. According to Marion Finkel, however, many of these are in early R&D stages and probably will not develop to the NDA stage.

Initially, Finkel had announced the FDA's intention to require that drugs intended for diseases prevalent in other nations but rare in the United States would have to affect at least 500 people in this country in order for the drug to be designated as an orphan. This was

Table 8–8
Drugs Designated by FDA as Orphans, as of June 1984

Generic Name[a]	Sponsor	Intended Use
Submitted from commercial sponsors		
Diaziquone	Warner–Lambert Co.	Brain malignancies
Alpha-1-antitrypsin (AAT)	Cooper Biomedical	AAT deficiency
Hexamethylmelamine (Hexastat)	Ives Laboratories	Ovarian carcinoma
Pentamidine isethionate	LyphoMed Inc.	Pneumocystis carinii pneumonia
L-Carnitine	American McGaw	Genetic carnitine deficiency
Cromolyn sodium (Cromoral)	Fisons Corp.	Mastocytosis
Bacitracin, U.S.P.	A.L. Laboratories, Inc.	Specific type of enterocolitis
Hemin (Panhematin)	Abbott Laboratories	Acute intermittent porphyria
Ethanolamine oleate	Glaxo, Inc.	Bleeding esophageal varices
Epoprostenol prostacyclin, PGI, PGX (Flolan)	Burroughs–Wellcome Co.	Heparin replacement
DMSA[b]	Johnson & Johnson	Lead poisoning in children
PEG-ADA[c] (Imudon)	Enzon, Inc.	Enzyme replacement therapy for ADA deficiency
Monooctanoin (Capmul 8210)	Ascot Pharmaceuticals, Inc.	Cholesterol gallstone dissolution
Viloxazine hydrochloride (Vivalan)	Stuart Pharmaceuticals	Narcolepsy and cataplexy
Clofazimine (Lamprene)	Ciba–Geigy Corp.	Leprosy resistant to Dapsone
Submitted by individual investigators		
Botulinum A toxin (Oculinum)	A.B. Scott, M.D. (San Francisco)	Strabismus and blepharospasm

Source: Adapted from "Orphan Drug Designations Thru June 1984," Orphan Designations Pursuant to Section 526 of the Orphan Drug Act (P.L. 97-414), June 30, 1984, #84N-0102.

[a]Trade names are in parentheses.
[b]2,3-dimercaptosuccinic acid.
[c]PEG-adenosine deaminase.

to guard against "subverting" the Act. The House report accompanying the bill, however, as discussed in the previous chapter, had indicated that to the extent the act facilitated efforts on behalf of drugs needed in other countries, this was in the public good. It might also alleviate a major obstacle for the Agency for International Development (AID) in providing drugs to other nations. Currently AID cannot directly supply developing nations with drugs that are not approved by the FDA. This is to protect countries against receipt of drugs that are *nonapproved* (those judged not to be safe and/or effective) as well as those that are simply *unapproved* (those that have not been reviewed for marketing by FDA). Often companies have been reluctant to incur FDA approval costs for drugs intended for developing nations, historically an unprofitable market. The Act might lessen this disincentive. Strong arguments in support of the limitation suggested by FDA would be needed before it would gain widespread public agreement. FDA is still considering the matter.

In the meantime, a more direct solution to the problem has been proposed by Senator Hatch in S. 2878. The bill would allow U.S. drug companies to sell unapproved new drugs to other nations. It would prohibit, however, exportation of drugs which have been banned in the United States, drugs which have not been approved by the importing countries, and drugs which are improperly labeled (those which exaggerate effective uses or which do not contain information on adverse effects). The FDA and World Health Organization support the bill.[8]

Under guidelines for implementing Section 525, whereby FDA is to provide recommendations for orphan-drug investigations, sponsors are to provide sixteen points of information, including—in addition to name of sponsor, generic and trade name of drug, and the like—details of the drug's development status, route of administration, and dosage form, all of which affect the type of review FDA would need to conduct. Other points of information required include: summary of pharmacologic effects, available nonclinical and clinical data, an outline of protocols under which the drug has been or is being studied and an interpretation of resulting data, a detailed plan for safety and efficacy studies, clinical trial protocols if available, and a list of specific questions FDA is to address in its recommendations for nonclinical and clinical studies. Additionally, financial information supporting the claim for orphan designation is required.

After receiving the information, FDA has 30 days to inform the sponsor of its decision on whether to give the application an orphan designation. Those that do qualify then will undergo review to determine the additional nonclinical and clinical studies FDA officials expect to be necessary for approval. This may include a meeting with the sponsor. Whether or not a meeting is held, written recommendations will be provided to the drug sponsor within 120 days from receipt of the initial application. Subsequent recommendations then will be based on data accumulated during early investigation of the drug, according to the guidelines.

Reportedly, the Patent and Trademark Office has agreed to expedite the patent review of orphan products, accelerating decisions so that FDA can determine whether seven-year market exclusivity applies. A memorandum of understanding to this effect, signed by FDA, appeared in the Federal Register on April 5, 1984.

As mentioned in the previous chapter, industry officials were critical of the Act's provision concerning tax credits and deductions for the cost of clinical trials. They contend that the major cost disincentive is ongoing toxicology and pharmacology studies, which are conducted concurrently with phase I and II clinical trials. The trials often are the least costly element, since relatively few numbers of patients are involved. The IRS has concluded that at least through 1987 the tax credit and deductions will not apply to preclinical work, including phase I and II toxicology. The rationale is that it is too difficult to separate and monitor nonclinical work undertaken on the orphan uses as opposed to the nonorphan uses of a given drug. The potential for abuse of the provision was considered to outweigh by far the countervailing argument. It is too early to evaluate what effect this strict interpretation of the tax provisions will have on industry drug development decisions. If, as one major drug company official commented, the industry would be involved in orphan drugs even in the absence of the current law, then the IRS decision may be accepted as a necessary limitation to tax benefits. The Treasury Department will issue the guidelines concerning the tax credit and market exclusivity provisions, but reportedly has been taking longer than expected to do so.

The potential of tax credits provided in the Recovery Tax Act of 1981 (discussed in Chapter 4) to stimulate industrial R&D in all fields, however, has been assessed preliminarily as less than many proponents had expected. An analysis conducted by the National Science Foundation and directed by University of Pennsylvania economist Edwin Mansfield suggests that increased R&D expenditures attributable to the 1981 Tax Act incentives seem to be substantially less than the corresponding government revenue loss. According to a recent article, John LaFalce (D-N.Y.), Chairman of the Subcommittee on Economic Stabilization of the House Banking Committee, said the study means that for every dollar of tax revenue lost, the country is gaining only a 30 cent increase in industrial R&D.[9] Mans-

186 • *Orphan Drugs*

field cautions, however, that several factors may confound pessi-
mistic conclusions. For instance, some of the 110 firms with major
R&D programs surveyed are not affected by the credits, some may
want to cut back R&D spending, and others may have no tax liability
against which to apply credits. Mansfield said that according to company officials, R&D is a small part of a large investment needed to
bring products to the market; therefore, R&D inducements have a
limited effect. It will be interesting to evaluate the effects of the
orphan-drug tax provision within this framework several years from
now.

The first recombinant DNA product to receive orphan status may
illustrate the IRS rationale. The drug is alpha-1 antitrypsin (AAT)
for hereditary emphysema, estimated to affect 54,000 people in the
United States. AAT is under development by CooperBiomedical Inc.
with two other corporate collaborators, one of which (Zymogenetics)
did the genetic engineering. Intravenous administration of AAT may
prevent damage to lungs caused by lack of the body's own supply of
the protein that ordinarily neutralizes the lung-damaging enzyme,
elactase. According to a CooperBiomedical official, however, the
company also plans to test AAT using another route of administration in other types, including emphysema occurring from smoke
inhalation in fire victims, and in chronic cigarette smokers. If AAT
is found to be effective for these uses, the drug's likely financial
return would equal the company's investment, according to the
CooperBiomedical official, whose estimate may be grossly conservative.[10]

By February 1984, FDA had industry commitments to sponsor
twenty-four orphan-drug products, some of which have been designated orphan under the law, and two of which have been approved
for marketing, as shown in Table 8–9. Additionally, FDA has provided an update on several of the drugs of limited commercial interest the agency identified during the 1981 orphan-drug hearings
(Table 8–10). The office has sought these sponsors through a number
of channels, including the PMA commission, the GPIA Institute for
Orphan Drugs, and publication in the Federal Register.[11]

In sum, it appears that FDA's net has, within a short period,
drawn in both present and future orphan drugs, taking the lead in
this latter category through grant awards, while the PMA and GPIA
still are trying to formulate policy for stimulating development of
new orphan products. However, the FDA still needs to develop a
systematic approach to informing clinical researchers about FDA's
potential review assistance and special review procedures, and to

Table 8–9
Sponsor Commitments for Orphan Products, Announced by FDA

Drug	Use	Sponsor
Commitments Made Before P.L. 97-414 (January 4, 1983)[a]		
Methacholine Cl	Bronchial asthma diagnosis	Roche
1-5HTP	Postanoxic myoclonus	Bolar
Amiodarone	Cardiac arrhythmias	Ives
Hematin[b,c]	Hepatic porphyria	Abbott
Trien	Wilsons Disease	Merck
NP-59	Adrenal cortical imaging	Mallinckrodt
Indium[111] Oxine	Platelet imaging	Amersham
Pimozide[b,c]	Tourette syndrome	McNeil
Bacitracin[b]	Pseudomembranous Enterocolitis	A.L. Laboratories
Hydroxy-ethyl starch	White blood cell harvesting	American Critical Care
Vitamin E	Neuromuscular disorders[d]	Roche
Pentamidine[b]	P. Carinii pneumonia	Zenith
Carnitine[b]	Carnitine deficiency	McGaw
Ethanolamine oleate[b]	Bleeding esophageal varices	Glaxo, Inc.
Confidential	—	—
Commitments Made After P.L. 97-414 signed[e]		
Lamprene[b]	Leprosy	Ciba-Geigy
Deprenyl	Parkinsons disease	Confidential
I[131] MIBG	Adrenal medullary imaging	Mallinckrodt
Monooctanoin[b]	Cholesterol gallstone dissolution	Ascot
Solution[f]	Urinary tract conditions	Guardian Chemical
Furamide	Asymptomatic intestinal amebiasis	Boots Pharm.
Mitronal	Hereditary angioneurotic edema	G.D. Searle
Confidential	—	—
Confidential	—	—

Source: Adapted in part from "Orphan Drugs and Devices Sponsor Commitments," prepared by FDA, presented to PMA commission, April 1984, and updated in June 1984. Also adapted from "Orphan Designations Pursuant to Section 526 of the Orphan Drug Act (P.L. 97-414) through June 30, 1984," #84N-0102.

[a]Still may be eligible for orphan designation under the law.

[b]Officially designated orphan under the law.

[c]Approved for marketing.

[d]Secondary to cholestatic disease in vitamin E–deficient patients.

[e]Eligible to be designated as orphan under the law.

[f]Citric acid, gluconic acid, magnesium hydroxycarbonate, magnesium acid citrate, calcium carbonate solution.

Table 8–10
Updates of Drugs of Little Commercial Interest,
Identified by FDA in 1981 Hearings

Drug	Current Status
Cobalt EDTA	Safer compound under study
P-chloro-1-phenylalanine	No longer considered orphan
I^{131} Norcholesterol	Mallinckrodt, Inc.[a]
Cyanoacrylate	NDA submitted, commercial sponsor
Sodium cellulose phosphate	NDA approved, Mission Pharmaceutical
Acetohydroxamic acid	NDA approved, Mission Pharmaceutical
Phenoxybenzamine	Commercial sponsor, IND available
2,3, Dihydroxybenzoic acid	More effective compound under study
NAPA	Commercial sponsor, studies underway
Physostigmine	Commercial sponsor, IND availability
Naltrexone	NDA submitted, DuPont
L3,4, dehydroproline	Research in progress
Trasylol	Commercial sponsor, studies underway
Keto/amino acids	Commercial sponsor, studies underway
Cytomel injection kit	SmithKline, available through IND
Sodium fluoride	Research in progress
LAAM	NIDA submitted an NDA, available as IND
Phosphocysteamine	Available as IND, GPIA, PMA funding study
Japanese B encephalitis vaccine	Available as IND
Hematin	NDA approved, Abbott
Amiodarone	IND, Ives
1-5HTP	IND, Bolar
Methacholine	IND, Roche

Source: Adapted in part from "Table 1: Current Status of Products of Limited Commercial Value" in Orphan Products Board 1982–1983 Annual Report; from Steven Groft, FDA, June 1984; and from "Sponsor Commitments for Orphan Products, FDA."

[a]From the PMA "Disposition of Formal Proposals Approved."

informing physicians about the Compassionate IND and Treatment IND mechanisms under which they can obtain orphan drugs. FDA also needs to evaluate whether current announcements of available grant funds are adequately reaching university scientists. Moreover, attention to coordinating FDA approval requirements with NIH drug development grantees seems essential to the success of stimulating orphan drug efforts by academia. Finally, it is anticipated that FDA will carefully evaluate on an ongoing basis its actions as drug project funder and approver. The entire area of FDA involvement in supporting drug development is new, although in the past several years the agency has assembled data for certain orphan candidates. On the one hand, it epitomizes the call by some in industry for FDA to balance its efforts to keep unsafe and ineffective drugs off the market while at the same time facilitating rapid market availability of those that are safe and effective. On the other hand, it confounds the agency's role as regulator with one as development funder. The necessity for FDA to communicate early with sponsors, as stipulated in the new law, may minimize the potential conflict-of-interest situation for FDA. If likely NDA requirements are spelled out by its officials prospectively, FDA should not be faced with making adverse rulings on drugs developed in part through agency grant support. Nonetheless, FDA will need to be aware of the consequences of its new dual role.

The $4 million annual appropriation authorization under the Orphan Drug Act for funding drug research has not been budgeted by OMB as of this writing. Consequently, no funds have been appropriated for this purpose by Congress and therefore no grants under this provision have been awarded. According to some industry officials, the sum is trivial; others say well-placed funding could be helpful. Since FDA received fifty-eight applications competing for the twelve grants awarded with the $500,000 Whitten amendment to the FDA appropriation, the Orphan Drug Act's annual $4 million fund is likely to be rapidly spent. Other questions have been raised: Can the research funds be applied to new products efficiently and effectively? Should direct federal funding for orphan-drug research be encouraged above that which NIH grants for orphan-drug projects? If so, who should coordinate the grant priorities between the NIH institutes and the DHHS Orphan Products Board, which ultimately would have authority over the $4 million grant awards?

The DHHS Orphan Products Board, of all the public and private groups, has been viewed as the most closed in its activities. Recently, PMA's Theodore Cooper convinced Assistant Secretary for Health Edward Brandt that closer communication between the two groups was essential to avoid duplication of efforts and to coordinate public- and private-sector actions.[12] Brandt agreed and designated Glenna Crooks of the board to serve as liaison to the PMA commission. Furthermore, he has formed a New Deal type of informal kitchen cabinet to promote discussions among major figures in orphan-drug planning efforts. The DHHS board has held at least one public meeting since its inception, and plans additional ones in the future.

According to the board's first annual report covering March 1982 to May 1983, members have become better informed of DHHS activities currently under way on orphan products, including those within several of the federal research institutes. It also has initiated discussion with the Health Care Financing Administration (HCFA) to determine policies for Medicare and—by example—Medicaid for reimbursement for orphan products in IND status.[13] In what may be circular reasoning, HCFA responded that IND drugs generally have not demonstrated safety and efficacy to the extent that NDA's have, and therefore are not appropriate candidates for reimbursement when compared to their marketed counterparts. The HCFA opinion does not take into consideration those marketed drugs for common diseases that do not have approved supplemental NDAs for use in rare diseases but instead are left in Compassionate IND status. These drugs are on the market and are bought by patients who have prescriptions for them but then cannot be reimbursed. HCFA also does not consider cases of Compassionate INDs that are judged by FDA to have sufficient safety and efficacy determinations to warrant their premarket distribution in the absence of marketed therapies, and that may not have NDAs because sponsors have not considered it cost-efficient to apply for them. Nor does it consider the similar case for Treatment INDs. Apparently most but not all drugs in these investigational categories are provided at no charge. The DHHS report indicates HCFA is willing to look at the issue on a case-by-case basis, but apparently no systematic method for reviewing the cases has been developed. Moreover, consumers are excluded from the DHHS Orphan Products Board's closed meetings. Yet they are most likely to be aware of and concerned about the reimbursement problem on specific cases. As FDA tries to systematize the Treatment IND program, closer coordination of FDA and HCFA decisions seems prudent.

The DHHS board also is considering the liability problem, according to its 1982–1983 report. Reportedly liability is a major concern to GPIA firms, which do not have self-insurance. Unlike most PMA firms, GPIA firms may lack the resources to weather a severe liability outcome. Also at issue, though not discussed in the report, is the considerable problem of liability faced by individual academic drug researchers, including those receiving federal grants. Liability barriers have negatively affected university sponsorship of orphan drugs, a substantial obstacle for academic scientists involved in orphan product development. These problems seem to warrant the full attention of the DHHS board.

Although the board has advised DHHS research agencies to flag grants involving orphan products as sensitive, the board has not taken the lead to date in coordinating NIH-FDA grant activities to avoid conflicting requirements, as mentioned earlier and as detailed by Upjohn President William Hubbard whose company found that submitting NCI data did not meet NDA application requirements.

Finally, there has been no apparent communication between the DHHS board and the office at NIH involved in awarding grants to small businesses. This is another area in which greater coordination may be useful.

It is still early in the board's life. Its potential for coordinating federal efforts and for interacting with industry is substantial. The outlook for better government-industry cooperation seems brighter since Cooper's overture to encourage greater communication between planners in the two sectors. Creative approaches to cooperation should at least be explored, and both industry and federal agency officials should use these organizations as referents. For instance, one suggestion for joint interaction with industry, suggested by Bert Spilker of Burroughs Wellcome Company, concerns information exchange. Spilker suggested his company would be in a better position to look into potential new orphan-disease products if the DHHS board indicated which ones currently have animal models. Where appropriate models exist, Spilker suggested the board also provide names of experts in those fields, and of voluntary organizations able to provide systematic networking for identifying possible clinical-trial participants. This is similar to the clearinghouse being developed by GPIA on a more limited scale and to a clearinghouse idea being explored by the board. Although the DHHS board has concluded that a listing of all known orphan diseases could be an enormous task with dubious payoff, providing information on diseases which do have animal models—if not already known to industry—could be potentially useful, as Spilker suggests.

Voluntary Agency Initiatives

The National Organization for Rare Disorders (NORD) formed in 1982 and headed by Ruby Horansky (executive director of the National Huntingtons Disease Association) has been a constant force in lobbying for public- and private-sector efforts for orphan products. The organization's liaison for government affairs, Abbey Meyers of the Tourett Syndrome Association, puts out a quarterly update report on the progress of those efforts, and members of the organization are frequent attendees at PMA commission meetings. Recently NORD presented awards for outstanding contributions to orphan-disease progress. Recipients included Representative Jamie Whitten, Marion Finkel of FDA, Max Linc of Sandoz, William Haddad of the GPIA, and Sydney Dworkin of Revco.

The National Drugs and Devices Foundation, headed by Joel Bennett, has been slow to develop but now appears to be gathering momentum. Initially, according to Bennett, the foundation expects to fund product-oriented R&D, but eventually may try to support basic research as well. Reportedly the FDA Office of Orphan Products Development will refer grant applications to the foundation for funding consideration from among those favorably reviewed by FDA's advisory council but not recieving any of FDA's limited grant awards. Bennett has emphasized that the foundation is neither obliged to fund applications recommended by FDA nor constrained in funding those that have not been reviewed or favorably endorsed by the FDA. It is not clear, however, on what other basis the foundation would make those decisions. Its board reflects a broad constituency, including Senator Nancy Kassebaum; Representative Henry Waxman; GPIA President Bill Haddad; Robins President E. Clairborne Robins, Jr.; Sandoz chairman Max Linc; Henry Schein, Inc. Chairman Jacob Schein; Jeffrey Martin Chariman Martin Himmel; and Burroughs Wellcome Chairman William Sullivan. Linc and Haddad are the executive committee's vice-chairmen.[14]

Unfinished Business and New Legislative Proposals

Besides evaluating current orphan-drug activities in terms of what is being done, it is instructive to evaluate plans in terms of what they omit or have not even considered. The Orphan Drug Act applies specifically to drugs and biologicals for rare diseases and conditions. As mentioned earlier, although Representative Waxman was well aware of the other types of problems conferring orphan status, the legislation was not meant to be a cure-all.

Lest problems of unpatentable drugs for larger populations or those of drugs with high liability risks (especially vaccines) be lost to follow-up, legislation concerning both issues has been under consideration by Congress. For instance Upjohn defines an orphan drug simply as one whose return on investment from sales does not equal costs, according to Jacob Stucki, an Upjohn vice-president for pharmacological research. It cannot be stated more clearly. Incidence or prevalence of a disease is a factor only to the extent it influences this equation. Equally important, he emphasized, was patentability of the drug and the cost of the basic material. These two factors, according to Stucki, are major determinants in drug development decisions. Where drugs for rare diseases have no patent protection, the seven-year market exclusivity may give the company breathing room, he said. But unpatentable drugs for larger markets have persistently encountered development obstacles. A new law (P.L. 98-417) to address that problem is part of a complicated strategy to balance the needs of GPIA companies with those of PMA companies.

For several years, Representative Waxman has advocated the need for legislation that would stimulate the generic drug industry. Through the Abbreviated NDA process (ANDA), generic manufacturers have been able to market generic forms of patented drugs approved before 1962 once those patents expired. However, no process has been instituted to allow generic companies similarly to market generic forms of such drugs approved since 1962. Conversely, the PMA has lobbied for some years to have restored to them the period of patent term which is used while drugs are undergoing FDA review. Waxman has combined these two issues into a single bill, which underwent more than twenty-five drafts because of its complexity and its need to satisfy both GPIA and PMA member firms. By formula, drugs whose NDAs are now submitted can be eligible to gain up to five additional years of patent protection at the time the drug's seventeen-year patent life expires. Drug NDAs under review at the time of passage of the law (September 24, 1984) can receive a two-year patent extension. The bill limits total post-marketing protection to fourteen years. Generic manufacturers would be able to market generic equivalents of drugs approved since 1962 at the time their patent expires. According to Haddad, there are about 120 such drugs with patents that already have expired. As part of the bill, drugs that are not patentable would enjoy a four-year period of market exclusivity during which time FDA would not approve ANDAs for generic equivalents. This provision is similar to the seven-year market exclusivity provision in the Orphan Drug Law, applying to unpatentable drugs for rare diseases. Since survey data indicate that several unpatentable drugs intended for large populations are considered orphans by both industry and federal agency sponsors, this provision may stimulate development of unpatentable drugs in general.

The second piece of proposed legislation concerns a program for compensation for the rare victims of adverse effects from vaccines. Introduced by Senator Paula Hawkins (R-Fla.), the National Childhood Vaccine-Injury Compensation Act (S. 2117) would enable victims to choose one of two avenues of compensation. One is the usual torts process, which is the way such claims currently are handled. Alternatively, the victim's parents could choose an administrative no-fault remedy. The bill establishes a revolving trust fund that initially could be established by Treasury loans which eventually would be repaid by a surcharge levied on vaccine manufacturers. Those who elect to pursue compensation through the fund would need to prove that they were vaccinated and subsequently (within a specified period of time) had an injury listed on the Vaccine Injury Table, and that they have not received compensation through the tort system. The bill also would set up recording and reporting mechanisms by health-care providers, and would instruct the DHHS secretary to study scientific reports of vaccine contraindications to attempt to identify high-risk populations and to study the relationship between vaccines and certain illnesses.

Vaccine manufacturers, including Wyeth, Lederle, Merck, and Connaught (a Canadian firm for which Squibb is the U.S. distributor), reportedly have insisted that the administrative remedy alone be offered, cutting off access to compensation through the torts system. The Trial Lawyers Association insists on availability of both avenues. In the meantime, Wyeth has announced it no longer will produce the controversial pertussis vaccine because of the increased liability costs, further reducing the seriously dwindling number of vaccine producers. Moreover, the bill does not address compensation for adults who suffer vaccine sequelae. The National Academy of Science's current study on a range of vaccine-related issues should be valuable in future efforts concerning this lingering public health dilemma. The bill introduced by Hawkins is an initial attempt to create a systematic policy. Comments on the legislation so far suggest there is a long way to go.

From National to International Action

The Orphan Drug Act of 1983 is confined within U.S. boundaries, with the exception of its potential to stimulate development of drugs little needed here but desperately needed in other nations. The tragic effects of disease, however, like multinational firms, are worldwide.

It is too early to tell what effect, if any, the Orphan Drug Act in the United States will have on international ethical drug directions. An indication may be the case of Ciba-Geigy, based in Switzerland. The company is readying an NDA for lamprene to be used in leprosy, whose U.S. incidence has increased 500 percent since 1960, to 5,000 people, primarily those emigrating here from Asian and Latin American countries. INDs for testing lamprene in other immunologic disorders, possibly AIDS and multiple sclerosis, also are contemplated. Notably, Ciba-Geigy has decided to provide lamprene to the Indian government to treat some 22,000 patients with leprosy on the condition that the government keeps the firm informed of details of its leprosy control program. In fact, Ciba-Geigy is said to be reducing the cost of three drugs recommended by the World Health Organization (WHO) for leprosy, thereby making them potentially more accessible to developing nations. concomitantly, Ciba-Geigy has initiated a program to look at drugs for other tropical diseases to see if they are appropriate for use on this country.[15]

Conversely, some other nations reportedly are considering whether to follow the U.S. lead and, if so, how, according to an article in the WHO bulletin. Attention focused on orphan drugs, the article emphasizes, brings pharmaceuticals for developing nations into sharp relief and underscores the need for directed research on that area of therapeutics.[16] The Japanese Council for Promotion of New Drugs now is investigating means for fostering orphan-drug development, according to recent reports.[17] The United Kingdom's Royal Society of Health held a June 1984 meeting in London on "Orphans of the World of Medicine."[18] The Swedish *Apoteksbolag* (ACL) has begun to compile a list of orphan drugs in Sweden and will attempt to build up a body of knowledge through documentation and research on about eighty substances intended for rare-disease use.[19] Finally, the legislation recently introduced by Senator Hatch to allow export of unapproved drugs to other nations may, if enacted, open the way for more attention by U.S. firms to drugs needed in the Third World. In the international arena, the world of orphan drugs meets the world of drugs for common diseases. It is a challenging juncture.

Notes

1. Eric Trist, "A Concept of Organizational Ecology: Invited Address, Melbourne Universities, 1976," *National Labor Union Bulletin* 12(1976): 483–496.
2. PMA Commission on Drugs for Rare Diseases, "Annual Report," 1982, pp. 1–12.
3. Kenneth Larsen, Zenith, personal communication, June 26, 1984.
4. "Accessing Rare Disease Information with your Personal Computer," *Generics*, Spring 1984, p. 16.
5. William Haddad, GPIA, presentation at Mt. Sinai Orphan Drugs Meeting, April 10, 1984.

6. Patrick Donoho, Revco, D.S. Inc., personal communication, June 26, 1984.

7. Stuart Nightingale, "Presentation to the PMA Commission on Drugs for Rare Diseases," February 18, 1982, pp. 1–6.

8. Joan Radovich, "FDA Backs Export of New Drugs," *Philadelphia Inquirer*, July 28, 1984, p. A02.

9. John Walsh, "Do Tax Credits for R&D Work?" *Science 224*(April 6, 1984):39.

10. Jeffrey L. Fox, "Gene-Splicing Protein to Have Orphan Status," *Science 223*(March 2, 1983):914.

11. "Annual Report: Activities of the Orphan Products Board," USPHS, DHHS, March 1982–May 1983, pp. 1–16.

12. PMA commission meeting minutes, June 2, 1983, p. 2.

13. "Annual Report."

14. *Drug Research Reports* (The Blue Sheet), March 21, 1984, p. P&R5.

15. *F-D-C Reports* (The Pink Sheet), April 16, 1984, pp. T&G3,4.

16. *Scrip*, April 9, 1984, p. 15.

17. *Scrip*, February 28, 1983, No. 772, p. 13.

18. *Scrip*, April 2, 1984, No. 884, p. 19.

19. *Scrip*, February 27, 1984, No. 874, p. 1.

9
Orphan Drug Planning: Larger Policy Implications

The task outlined in Chapter 1 was to see where we stood with orphan drugs. In Chapter 9 the task is to consider whether the planning processes and policies developed for dealing with orphan drugs hold any implications for the larger system of which they are a part—namely, therapeutics—and for the many problems faced in the health-care arena. As a means of summarizing the first task, perhaps a follow-up of examples presented in Chapter 1 will convey a general sense of the situation.

Melvin Van Woert has found a generic drug firm (Bolar) that is undertaking sponsorship of L-5HTP for treating patients with myoclonus, as a result of the efforts of the GPIA Institute on Orphan Drugs.

John Walshe has found a willing sponsor for trien, the drug that probably has saved the life of his nine-year-old patient with Wilsons disease and others like him. Merck, as a result of the process set out by the PMA Commission on Drugs for Rare Diseases, is sponsoring the NDA.

The Health Care Financing Administration (HCFA) began to reimburse patients hospitalized for ACTH therapy for multiple sclerosis after a university researcher presented data to FDA, securing the agency's approval for this orphan use of the widely marketed drug. But no systematic means has been developed for determining which—if any—marketed drugs labeled for use in common diseases, but also used for rare diseases, should be reimbursible.

The CDC has emergency supplies of the drug pentamidine to treat AIDS patients. This has been facilitated by efforts of the GPIA to guarantee supplies from the drug's British manufacturer until PMA-member LyphoMed develops and gains FDA approval for U.S. manufacture of the drug. The CDC may be able to avoid such crises in the future by contacting the PMA commission and the GPIA institute for assistance in similar situations.

Those providing public health care in the Third World may receive some assistance if the Orphan Drug Act stimulates increased development of drugs rarely needed in the United States but desperately needed in poorer countries. However, solutions for this and most other health-care problems in developing nations have not yet been found.

Federal research agencies continue to work on development of anticancer and other orphan drugs. If current orphan drug planning and policies serve to increase industry's role, the need for additional or even continued federal efforts may decrease. Greater federal agency coordination may be achieved through efforts of the DHHS Orphan Products Board; but basic issues remain to be addressed, such as whether to provide increased funding for drug R&D and, if so, where that funding will come from. Additionally, patent rights, trade-secret status of data, and liability issues are not yet well defined. Even so, the Orphan Products Board does provide a central organization through which FDA and NIH can coordinate drug development and approval activities, and through which these government agencies can plan interactively with industry firms and with the PMA commission and the GPIA institute.

Pharmaceutical firms have expressed a commitment to increase industry efforts on behalf of orphan drugs, although it is too early to tell whether the market and regulatory provisions of the new law will aid their efforts in a measurable way.

Finally, certain patients participating in a clinical trial of a newly marketed drug for parkinsonism are being provided the drug free of charge by its sponsor, Sandoz, according to University of Pennsylvania neurologist Howard Hurtig, who interceded in the patients' behalf. Most of these patients otherwise would not be able to afford the drug because of its astronomically high price of about $300 per month per patient; this price reflects the drug's high R&D costs. The solution described in this particular instance is temporary and limited; the problem itself is constant and widespread. The example brings us to a final question that orphan drug planners and policymakers have not really addressed: Should orphan drugs be developed regardless of cost? If not, who will decide where to draw the line? In either case, who will pay?

Explicitly predetermined answers to these questions are not likely to be forthcoming; rather, the answers will be enunciated piecemeal and implicitly through future behavior of industry, government, and health-care consumers of both orphan and nonorphan drugs. Rapid technological advances in drugs or other medical therapies may change the medical environment to such an extent that the questions that are obvious today are obsolete tomorrow.

One of the tools of systems analysis is the use of the dialectic, the Hegelian method of forging a synthesis between the thesis (a proposition defended in argument) and its antithesis (an opposing proposition). *Dialectic* comes from the Greek *dialektikos*, meaning "conversation." For the first time in orphan-drug policy and planning, mechanisms exist for constituent groups, each with its own set of views on the issues, to converse *with* one another about policies instead of talking *at* one another through the press and scientific journals. It will be interesting to see whether these new forums will address the fundamental questions that remain, such as the classic one of whether to use limited resources to develop drugs needed by many or drugs needed by a few. The creative aspect of dealing with this dilemma is changing the *or* to an *and* relationship. Unlike the guns-or-butter analogy, development of rare and common disease drugs needs not be mutually exclusive. Creation of new, innovative approaches to aid development of drugs in both categories is already underway. In part this may be achieved through technological advances that enable drug development at lower cost. In part it may be achieved by greater coordination in efforts to test and approve drugs developed by industry, government, and academia. In part it may be achieved by dissolution of regulatory obstacles to drug approval by improving on that system. In part it may be achieved through financial incentives specifically for orphan drugs, such as those contained in the current Orphan Drug Act and by direct fundraising such as that of the recently created National Foundation for Orphan Drugs, on whose board sit representatives from several of the different stake-holder groups, including industry and Congress. Orphan-drug development may also be aided by greater collaboration between PMA and GPIA firms, and academia, such as the current undertaking by one PMA member and two GPIA member firms on development of zinc therapy by an academic scientist. These are only a beginning, but at least the dialogue and the interactive planning process has begun.

The basic dilemmas posed by orphan drugs are the same as those posed by other new but expensive medical technologies being developed and introduced at a time of unprecedented escalations in health-care costs. These include surgical innovation such as transplants for hearts, livers, and kidneys, and heart implants. They also include other, nonsurgical innovations, of which kidney dialysis is the best-known example. The public cannot afford to ignore questions of which patients should receive the benefits of these advances, who should decide, and who should pay for them. The frequent practice of television newscasters appealing for donations for the latest child tragically affected by a diseased liver and in need of money for an experimental transplant will not assure the long-term viability of effective liver transplantation programs.[1] For instance, the possibility has just barely been addressed of whether health insurers might cover some of the costs of experimental trials, both medical and surgical, to determine efficacy. Funds spent prospectively might save money for insurers—and, by extension, the public—in the long run, if those deemed ineffective are no longer reimbursed.[2]

Russell Ackoff of the Wharton School, one of the major figures in the development of the systems approach to societal problems, emphasizes the need to solve problems not by taking them apart but by viewing them as part of a larger problem and by then making changes in the larger system. Those behaving in accordance with systems theory use ends (or goals) that are achieved as the means to reach the next end, in an ever-enlarging process. Ackoff emphasizes the opportunity for society, through this process, to redesign the future.[3] For patients with rare diseases whose lives have been affected by recent orphan-drug planning and policies, the future is being redesigned. If one doubts whether the system actually can work this way, ask the parents of the nine-year-old boy with Wilsons disease.

Notes

1. John K. Iglehart, "Health Policy Report: The Politics of Transplantation," *New England Journal of Medicine* 310(13)(1984):864–868.

2. Thomas C. Chalmers, Stanley van den Nort, Michael Lockshin, and Byron H. Waksman, "Special Report: Summary of a Workshop on the Role of Third-Party Payers in Clinical Trials of New Agents," *New England Journal of Medicine* 309(201)(1983):1334–1336; C. Ronald Kahn, "Sounding Board: A Proposed New Role for the Insurance Industry in Biomedical Research Funding," *New England Journal of Medicine* 310(4)(1984):257–258.

3. Russell Ackoff, *Redesigning the Future* (New York: Wiley, 1974).

Glossary of Abbreviations

AAT   alpha-1-antitrypsin, a drug under study for treatment of hereditary emphysema of the lung

ACTH   Adrenocorticotropic hormone, a substance occurring naturally in the body

ADAMHA   Alcohol, Drug Abuse and Mental Health Administration, a federal agency that is part of DHHS (see DHHS)

ADD   Antiepileptic Drug Development, a special program of NINCDS (see NINCDS)

AID   Agency for International Development, an executive branch federal agency

AIDS   Acquired Immune Deficiency Syndrome

ANDA   Abbreviated New Drug Application, used for FDA approval of a generic form of a drug marketed prior to 1962

CDC   Centers for Disease Control, a federal agency of DHHS involved in research and epidemiological surveillance of infectious and parasitic diseases, based near Atlanta, Georgia

CEO   Chief executive officer

Compassionate IND   An IND granted by FDA to allow interim use of an unapproved but medically needed drug still under investigation

DES   diethylstilbesterol, a synthetic female hormone

DHEW   Department of Health, Education and Welfare, former name of DHHS (see DHHS)

DHHS   Department of Health and Human Services, cabinet-level agency of the executive branch

DNA   deoxyribose nucleic acid, the strands of helically wound simple chemicals that make up the genetic material in the nucleus of every (eukaryotic) cell

FDA   Food and Drug Administration, a federal agency within DHHS responsible for drug approval

FTC   Federal Trade Commission, an executive branch federal agency

FY	Fiscal year
GAO	General Accounting Office, the congressional watchdog office
GBS	Guillain-Barré syndrome, an acute, often fulminant paralytic neurological disorder
GPIA	Generic Pharmaceutical Industry Association, a trade association
HCFA	Health Care Financing Administration, a federal agency of DHHS, which administers Medicare
IND	Notice of Claim for Investigational Exemption of a New Drug, an application that must be approved by FDA before a drug can be tested in humans
IRS	Internal Revenue Service, a division of the Treasury Department
LAAM	L-alpha-acetylmethadol, a drug under study as one alternative for methadone programs for former heroin addicts
MAC	Maximum Allowable Cost, a Medicare drug reimbursement program
FFDCA	Federal Food, Drug and Cosmetic Act
MIT	Massachusetts Institute of Technology
NASA	National Aeronautics and Space Administration
NCE	New chemical entity
NCI	National Cancer Institute, the largest of the NIH institutes
NDA	New Drug Application, an application submitted to FDA containing information required for approval of a new drug
NEI	National Eye Institute, part of NIH (see NIH)
NHLBI	National Heart, Lung and Blood Institute, part of NIH (see NIH)
NIAAA	National Institute on Alcohol and Alcohol Abuse, a division of ADAMHA
NIAID	National Institute of Allergy and Infectious Diseases, part of NIH
NIAMDDK	National Institute of Arthritis, Metabolic and Digestive Diseases and Kidney, part of NIH
NICHD	National Institute of Child Health and Human Development, part of NIH
NIDA	National Institute on Drug Abuse, a division of ADAMHA

NIH	National Institutes of Health, an agency of DHHS composed of several institutes
NIMH	National Institute of Mental Health, part of ADAMHA
NINCDS	National Institute of Neurological and Communicative Disorders and Stroke, part of NIH
NORD	National Organization for Rare Disorders, a voluntary agency consortium recently founded and located in New York City
NSF	National Science Foundation
OMB	Office of Management and Budget, an executive branch office
l-5HTP	l-5-hydroxy-tryptophan, a simple compound under study in the treatment of a rare neurological disorder, postanoxic myoclonus
OTA	Office of Technology Assessment, an office of the legislative branch
PHS	Public Health Service
P.L.	Public Law
PMA	Pharmaceutical Manufacturers Association, trade association for ethical (prescription) drug firms
R&D	Research and development
ROI	Return on investment
UCSD	University of California, San Diego
WHO	World Health Organization, based in Geneva, Switzerland

Index

About the Author

Carolyn H. Asbury, who received her undergraduate education in science and journalism, worked for several years as a science writer at the National Institutes of Health. She then completed a master's degree in public health at the Johns Hopkins School of Hygiene and Public Health, where she began research on orphan drugs. She completed the Ph.D. in social systems sciences at the Wharton School, University of Pennsylvania, where she specialized in health systems planning and policy. While at Wharton, she worked for the Busch Center, a consulting arm of the research department, where she did consulting in both the public and private sectors. Also during this time, she worked as an invited (unpaid) consultant to the Subcommittee on Health and the Environment, U.S. Congress, and to the Pharmaceutical Manufacturers Association Commission on Drugs for Rare Diseases.

After completing her degree, she was a postdoctoral research fellow at the University of California, San Francisco, Institute for Health Policy Studies, where she began this book, which she completed while a senior fellow at the Leonard Davis Institute of Health Economics at the University of Pennsylvania.

Dr. Asbury, who has published in the field of drug policy, now works at the Robert Wood Johnson Foundation of Princeton, New Jersey.